AF879048

BLOOD CHEMISTRY & CLINICAL NUTRITION

A MANUAL FOR THE PRACTICING HEALTH PROFESSIONAL

by Jack Tips, PhD, CCN

© 1993 by Jack Tips.

All rights reserved. No part of this discourse may be reproduced in any form without permission in writing from the publisher, Apple-A-Day Press.

Printed in the United States of America

Dr. Jack Tips, N.D. Ph.D., C.C.N., CHom
Life Resources / Apple-A-Day Natural Health Services
1500 Village West Drive, Suite 77
Austin, Texas 78733
Phone (512) 328-3996 • Fax (512) 263-7787
e-mail: apple-a-day@austin.rr.com
www.apple-a-daypress.com

This information is presented in good will for informational and educational purposes only.
All rights regarding the publishing of ths material are owned by Life Resources, Austin, Texas.

Contributing Editors:
Mr. Timothy Kuss
Dr. Robert Marshal

Layout & Design:
Andrew Carpenter

Proofreading:
Janine Tips

ISBN 0-929167-07-4
Library of Congress Catalog Card Number 93-73977

Systemic Formulas©, Systemic Formulas, Inc. Ogden, UT. Used with permission.

The products and product information presented in this discourse are in no way intended for use as a diagnostic tool, nor as a basis for prescribing: These are the responsibility of the health professional. This information is solely for educational reflection.

Date of Issue: November 1993

TABLE OF CONTENTS

HOW TO USE THIS MANUAL

BLOOD TESTS

ADDITIONAL INFORMATION

Blood Chemistry & Clinical Nutrition

Foreword

This manual is designed to help the health professional better understand the nutritional implications of blood chemistry and more effectively apply the Systemic Herbal Formulas to meet the nutritional and metabolic requirements of each individual's unique biochemistry.

Systemic Formulas have proven themselves to be a superior therapy to help correct metabolic and biochemical imbalances because they are designed to work specifically with the body tissues and systems responsible for maintaining health. When the glands and organs can function optimally, the automatic and impartial effect is a trend toward biochemical balance. Thus, the Systemic approach is to work with the body, the way the body was designed to work, and promote balance - bioenergetically, biochemically, and metabolically.

Three Keys to Success

Success in clinical nutrition means that you are effective in helping people excperience better health as a result of your evaluation and recommendations. To be successful as a clinical nutritionist, you need three things. First, are windows of insight to the **cause** of a person's symptoms. Second, is the ability to interpret the true meaning of the windows of insight. Thirdly, you need therapies that are safe, effective, and address the tissue or body-systems that are responsible for correcting the perceived imbalances.

For blood chemistry and clinical nutrition, the primary window of insight to the individual's health is the SMAC-26/CBC blood test with urinalysis plus other blood tests. From the blood values, the health professional is able to ascertain areas where the body is struggling to maintain homeostasis. Within the parameters of what the blood can reveal in a health profile survey (SMAC-26/CBC), deep insights can be gained regarding specific nutritional requirements so the body's specific systems can be nourished to experience better health. The clinical nutritionist may use several other modalities to gain an overview about a person's health status, but this manual will focus on blood tests.

The ability to interpret the true meaning of the blood values comes from a study of clinical nutrition and a lifetime commitment to understand the deep mysteries of the body and health. The International and American Association of Clinical Nutrition is the foremost organization to establish a course of training, certification exam, and continuing education regarding the interpretation of blood values and applications of clinical nutrition. By comparing the blood-test values from a lab report, the clinical nutritionist gains many insights on how to design an effective nutritional program to support whole-body health.

Once the insights gained from the interpretation of the blood values are organized into a well-thought-out plan of action, the next determining factor in successful work is effective tools. Many clinical nutritionists have found that Systemic Formulas add a greater dimension to their practices.

Briefly, Systemic Formulas were designed by A. S. "Doc" Wheelwright to provide nutritional support to balance whole body systems. For example, a person with blood values showing a hyper function of the adrenal cortex could benefit from the balancing effect the herbs and nutrients of the Ga-Adrenal formula. As the adrenal tissue, and other imbalances of the endocrine system, become more balanced due to the body's correction of the cause of the imbalance, the blood chemistry is able to reflect more optimal values. These changes are genuine changes reflective of the body's ability to correct its imbalances and strengthen its tissues when given the proper therapy.

Thus, the point here is that many health professionals have found the incorporation of Systemic Formulas into a nutrition regimen can bring the success as evidenced by deeper, more long-lasting results. This manual provides general guidelines for determining the appropriate nutritional support for each individual.

Best wishes in your blood chemistry endeavors.

How To Use This Manual

CUSTOM DESIGN THIS INFORMATION FOR YOUR INDIVIDUAL USE!

This manual is designed to be a reference tool for daily use. The lab tests are arranged alphabetically. For the most practical use, you should rearrange the pages in the order the lab tests appear on your lab report. This way you can flip through these pages in the order they appear on your lab's report. Since labs vary in the order they present information, you can custom-arrange this material to suit your needs. Now you have easily accessible information arranged to follow your blood report.

Here is a brief discussion of the information in each heading of each test.

The Optimal (Clinical Nutrition) Values - provides the numeric range that is optimal for overall body health. If a test value is either higher or lower than optimal, it should be considered as a significant insight regarding overall well-being of your patient. The optimal values are a much tighter range than the lab reference values.

The Pathological (Lab) Reference Values - provide the numeric range that Medicine has established as acceptable. If a test value is either higher or lower than that range, be alerted to potential pathological issues. Lab reference values vary from lab to lab depending on their population sample. If the lab you use bases its tests on different ranges just pencil them in.

The Definition And Discussion Of The Test - provides a brief explanation of the background and significance of the test, as well as any important clinical considerations.

Pathological Considerations - lists common pathologies associated with either increased or decreased test values. Increased values are higher than the Pathological (Lab) Reference Value. Decreased values are lower than the Pathological (Lab) Reference Value. The symbols to the right of the Pathological Considerations are formula codes for Systemic Formulas that can contribute to the body's efforts to correct such a concern.

Note: many of the diseases listed in this section are life-threatening and must be referred to qualified physicians. The listing of herbal formulas here does not make a claim that they can cure a disease. They are listed to support the body in its healing endeavors.

Clinical Nutrition - lists the Systemic nutritional supplements that have proven effective for correcting the increased or decreased test value. The formulas listed <u>in</u> the shaded boxes are the primary or first-thought-of formulas for general use. The formulas listed <u>under</u> the shaded boxes are secondary formulas to be considered to assist the primary formulas in comprehensive nutritional support. The italic nutrients are other recommendations, not currently manufactured by Systemic, but of value to the practice of clinical nutrition.

It is not uncommon for the same nutritional supplement to be indicated for both increased and decreased lab values. This is a testimony to the philosophy that clinical nutrition is a therapy that assists the body to balance its functions.

Clinical Cross-reference - lists the interrelated tests for a more complete evaluation of a specific health concern. Arrow Up (↑) is the abbreviation for an increased test value. Arrow Down (↓) is the abbreviation for a decreased test value. The equals sign (=) is the symbol for "consider or rule out the following concern." All test abbreviations are for serum values unless otherwise specified, i.e. "*Plasma Renin*".

Related Tests - provides other blood tests that confirm or enhance understanding of what the proper interpretation should be.

Clinical Notes - provides pertinent information regarding various issues about the specific test and its interpretation.

Warning - any test value that indicates a potentially life-threatening situation or disease process is listed here. It is essential for the clinical nutritionist to refer people with such values to medical expertise.

Practitioner Notes - Insights from experienced clinical nutritionists are listed here. After each insight, the contributors initials are given:

T.K.	=	Timothy Kuss
R.M.	=	Dr. Robert Marshal
J.T.	=	Jack Tips

Other Notes: Write down facts and insights that are important to your ability to interpret the specific test values and apply therapy.

Blood chemistry is a dynamic science. Changes to our understanding and applications of blood values occur regularly, due to the invention and initialization of newer and more specific blood tests and rediscovery of older tried-and-true tests. Contact the publisher, Apple-A-Day Press for updates to your manual. See the copyright page for the date of issue of your manual. If it has been over a year, there may be new information.

Blood Tests

ALBUMIN

Optimal (Clinical Nutrition) Values 4.7 - 5.2 g/dl.

Pathological (Lab) Reference Values: 3.5 - 5.5 g/dl.

Albumin: is a globular protein important to the maintenance of colloid osmotic pressure between arterial and venous capillaries and thus controls edema. It also transports vitamins, waste products, hormones such as thyroxin and cortisol, amino acids, and minerals including calcium and magnesium. It is the chief transport system for virtually everything in the body. Adequate Albumin levels are absolutely essential to the immune system. Albumin represents 60% of the total plasma protein and is produced in the liver.

Pathological Considerations:

Increased Albumin	
Dehydration	MIN
Hypothyroidism	Gf, #1, Gb
Lymphatic congestion	SENG

Decreased Albumin	
Anemia, pernicious	BSV, BLDB
Biliary cirrhosis	Lb, OXCC, OXAA, # 6
Cholecystitis, acute	Lb, Ls, #3
Congestive heart failure	H, PTM, EZV, Hcv
Dehydration	MIN
Digestive inflammation	D, #3, GOLD, AO, DCSU
Eclampsia	Nc, N3, K, L
Edema in extremities	KDIR, K, DSIR
Hypertension, essential	HCV, Ks
Hypochlorhydria	D, MIN
Liver disease, acute	L, Ls, #3, #4
Malnutrition (low protein)	PRO, D, MIN, AZV
Multiple sclerosis	Hn, OXCC, CAL, EZV, FLX
Nephritis, acute	K, #3, GOLD, ACX ACP
Nephrosis	K, Ks, #3
Portal cirrhosis	Lb, OXCC, OXAA, # 6
Pregnancy	L, BLDB
Renal dysfunction, extra vascular protein loss	K, Ks, #6, DSIR
Rheumatoid arthritis	ARTA, SENG, #3, Gt, WO

Clinical Nutrition:

For Increased Albumin	
LEV	Lecithin
Ps	Pancreas Stabilizer
BSV	Stress B-Vitamin

Di-Methyl Glycine

For Decreased Albumin	
LEV	Lecithin
D	Digestive
L	Liver

Gf Thyroid
BSV Stress B Vitamin
BLDB Blood Builder
Dl-Methionine
Zinc
Niacinamide
Chloride

Clinical Crossreference:

- **Albumin Depressed Due To Liver Dysfunction** = ↓ Albumin + alt. SGPT + Alt. GGTP
- **Congestive Heart Failure** = ↓ Albumin + ↑ SGOT + ↑ LDH
- **Digestive Inflammation** = ↓ Albumin + ↓ Globulin
- **Edema In Extremities** = ↓ Albumin + ↓ Total Protein
- **Hyperthyroidism** = ↓ Albumin + ↑ T3 Uptake (See T3 Uptake)
- **Kidney Stress** = ↓ Albumin + ↑ BUN (See Creatinine)
- **Liver Disease, Acute** = ↓ Albumin + ↑ SGOT + ↑ GGTP (See SGOT)
- **Protein Malnutrition & Liver Damage Suspected** = ↓ Albumin + ↓ BUN
- **Protein Malnutrition** = ↓ Albumin + ↓ Total Protein
- **Rheumatoid Arthritis** = ↓ Albumin + ↑ Alk. Phos. (See Alk. Phos.)

Related Tests:

A/G Ratio, Alkaline Phosphatase, BUN/Creatinine Ratio, Globulin, GGTP, Glucose, LDH, Protein Electrophoresis, SGOT, Uric Acid.

Clinical Notes:

- Albumin is considered by many health professionals to be the most reliable and scientific measure of good health.
- A decreased Albumin occurs in pregnancy.
- A lowered Albumin can be compensated by a rise in immunoglobins.
- If albumin is normal, it is difficult to detect any indicative rise in immunoglobins in Total Protein.

- The liver is the primary organ for protein synthesis. A weak liver usually will cause a lowered albumin.

- Bromsulphalein, a chemical dye that is injected into the bloodstream to test the liver's ability to remove it, (BSP test), will cause a false elevation of Albumin and Serum Protein. Wait three days after a BSP test before doing a blood test in such a case.

Practitioner Notes:

- Rapid rise of Albumin above 5.2 usually is associated with critical phases of illness. - R.M.

- Albumin decreases with the aging process making a person more susceptible to illness. - R.M.

- One or two tenths increase in Albumin can have a more profound benefit on the metabolism of calcium than any supplement yet known. - R.M.

- To correct a decreased albumin, be sure to improve hygiene. Do not use deodorant soaps. Also be sure the nail beds are clean. - R.M.

- A high Albumin is generally indicative of increased blood volume with toxic accumulation, lymphatic congestion, dehydration increased osmotic pressure and poor nutrient utilization. - J.T.

- A low Albumin is generally indicative of stress with collagen or vascular inflammation. - J.T.

Other Notes:

ALBUMIN/GLOBULIN RATIO (A/G RATIO)

Optimal (Clinical Nutrition) Values 1.5 - 2.0

Pathological (Lab) Reference Values: 1.1 - 2.5

Albumin/Globulin Ratio: Is the Albumin divided by Globulin. The optimal level is two parts albumin to one part Globulin. Of the three blood plasma proteins, Albumin, Globulin, and Fibrinogen, the A/G Ratio compares the two that maintain the colloidal osmotic pressure between plasma and tissue fluids. If Albumin and Globulin are low, tissue edema (water retention) often occurs as a result of the lowered osmotic pressure in the capillaries. Albumin is the most abundant plasma protein. Globulin is made up of Alpha 1, Alpha 2, Beta and Gamma. It is known that Albumin and Fibrinogen are synthesized in the liver, and most likely so is Globulin. Thus, liver disease can reduce the plasma proteins.

Since the A/G Ratio is not diagnostically specific, it is best compared to individual Albumin, Globulin, and Total Protein tests.

Pathological Considerations:

Increased Alb/Glob Ratio	
Hepatitis, infectious (also decreased)	L, GOLD, VIVI
Multiple myeloma (also decreased)	OXCC, OXAA, #5
Thyroid dysfunction	Gf, Gb

Decreased Alb/Glob Ratio	
Anemia, pernicious	BSV, BLDB, MIN
Hepatitis, infectious	L, GOLD, VIVI
Hypoproteinemia	PRO, D, MIN
Infections, chronic	#3, ATAK, Gt
Liver dysfunction	L, Ls, #5, #6
Lupus, erythematosus	OXCC, OXAA, #5, GT, S
Multiple myeloma	OXCC, OXAA, OXOX, #5
Nephritis	K, #3, GOLD
Nephrosis	K
Rheumatoid Arthritis	ARTA, SENG, #3, WO

Clinical Nutrition:

For Increased Alb/Glob Ratio

D Digestive
Gf Thyroid
LEV Lecithin

Ps Pancreas Stabilizer
L Liver Builder
FLX Flax Seed Oil
Vitamin A

For Decreased Alb/Glob Ratio

S Spleen
PRO Nutro Protein
K Kidney
L Liver

EZV Vitamin E 200
Gf Thyroid
Gt Thymus
Ls Liver Stimulant
Vitamin T (Sesame Seed Oil)

Clinical Crossreference:

- **Blood Clotting** = ↑ A/G Ratio
- **Blood, Too Thin (Lack of Fibrinogen and Tendency To Bleed)** = ↓ A/G Ratio
- **Hepatitis** = Altered A/G Ratio + ↑ SGOT + ↑ SGPT + ↑ WBC + ↑ Bilirubin
- **High Protein, High Caloric Diet** = ↑ A/G Ratio + ↑ Protein + ↑ Cholesterol
- **Liver Dysfunction** = ↓ A/G Ratio + ↑ GGTP + ↑ SGPT (See GGTP)
- **Protein Malnutrition** = ↓ A/G Ratio + ↓ Total Protein (See Total Protein)
- **Thyroid Dysfunction** = ↑ A/G Ratio + Altered T3 Uptake (See T3 Uptake)

Related Tests:

Albumin, Alkaline Phosphatase, BUN, BUN/Creatinine Ratio, Calcium, CBC, CEA, Creatinine, Globulin, GGTP, Glucose, LDH, Phosphohexose-Isomerase, Protein, SGOT, SGPT, Uric Acid, WBC.

Clinical Notes:

- A "low", "reversed", or "inverse" A/G Ratio suggests possible ulcerative colitis, intestinal obstructions, burns, peritonitis, chronic glomerulo-nephritis, portal cirrhosis, multiple myeloma, sarcoidosis, metastatic carcinoma, nephrotic syndrome, viral hepatitis, diabetic ketosis, severe thyrotoxicosis, untreated pernicious anemia, severe infections, cachexia, or congestive heart failure.

- Albumin is the body's transportation system. Specific binding proteins transport vitamins, minerals, fats, bilirubin, minerals and hormones throughout the body.

- Since albumin decreases in pregnancy, the A/G Ratio will also decrease.

Practitioner Notes:

- The key to all the proteins (albumin and the globulins) is the liver. Protein metabolism and protein synthesis are liver functions. Therefore, altered albumin and globulin and their ratios are often easily corrected with liver support. - J.T.

- A high A/G Ratio is generally indicative of <u>decreased</u> blood viscosity, impaired lymphatic circulation, and excessive toxicity. - J.T.

- A decreased A/G Ratio is generally indicative of increased blood viscosity and inflammation. - J.T.

Other Notes:

ALKALINE PHOSPHATASE (Alk. Phos.)

Optimal (Clinical Nutrition) Values 60 - 80 u/l

Pathological (Lab) Reference Values: 30 - 115 u/L

Childhood Reference Values:

0 - 9 years: 114 - 300 u/L

10 - 14 years: male: 105 - 380; female: 58 - 293 u/L

15 - 19 years: male: 47 144; female: 35 - 109 u/L

Lab ranges may vary due to different populations measured

Alkaline Phosphatase: Is an enzyme found primarily in the liver, bone, placenta, and intestinal mucosa. Its normal function is to facilitate hydrolysis of monophosphate at a pH of 9 - 10. When liver cells are damaged, or bone is rapidly growing (either normally or abnormally), or there are problems with the intestinal mucosa, large amounts of Alk. Phos. are released into the bloodstream. Thus, Alk. Phos. is used as a tumor marker as well as for insights regarding liver disease. In children, elevated Alk. Phos. is normal due to the rapid development of bone tissue.

The three primary tissues with a high content of Alk. Phos. can be identified individually by their isoenzymes. ALP-1 is formed in the liver and gall bladder. ALP-2 is derived from osteoblast cell activity of bone. ALP-3 is the isoenzyme produced by the intestinal mucosa. Regarding bone disease, since osteoblast cell involvement is required for ALP-2 increase, a pure bone lesion without osteoblast activity will not elevate ALP-2. Thus, Alk. Phos. is valuable for differential diagnosis of bone disease.

Decreased Alk. Phos. often occurs when there is a deficiency of zinc.

Pathological Considerations:

Increased Alkaline Phosphatase	
Adrenal cortex hyperfunction	Ga, #6, Gb
Birth control pills, steroids	L, Ls, Ga
Boeck's sarcoid	OXCC, #5, OXAA
Brucellosis	#3, GOLD, VIVI, ATAK
Cancer, liver	L, Ls, OXCC, #5, OXAA
Carcinoma of bone	OXAA, OXCC, #5, CTV
Chronic alcoholism	L, Ls, LEV, BSV
Cirrhosis, liver	L, Ls, OXCC, OXAA
Congestive heart failure	H, PTM, EZV
Diseases of the bone (osteoblastic activity)	OXAA, #5
Fragilitas ossium	CAL, MIN, *(magnesium)*
Hepatitis	L, GOLD, #4
Hodgkin's disease	OXCC, S, #5, OXAA
Hyperparathyroidism	Gf, #5
Hyperthyroidism	Gf, Gb, #5, L, Ls
Liver abscesses, disease	L, Ls, DSIR, #6, #3
Mononucleosis	L, Ls, GOLD, VIVI
Multiple myeloma	OXAA, OXCC, #5, K

continued

Decreased Alkaline Phosphatase	
Anemia	BLDB, MIN, BSV
Anemia, folic acid	BSV, AZV, BLDB, MIN
Celiac disease	D, P, AZV, MIN, DSIR, AO, DS
Cretinism	Gf, Gb, B, MIN
Hypochlorhydria	D, MIN, #1, Ds
Hypoparathyroidism	Gf, Gb
Hypophosphatasia	PRO
Hypothyroidism	Gf, #1, Gb, MIN
Nephritis, severe chronic	K, #3, ACX
Osteolytic sarcoma	OXAA, OXCC, #5
Protein malnutrition	PRO, D, Ds
Scurvy	CTV
Sexual precocity in children	CAL
Vitamin B-6 deficiency	BSV, AZV
Vitamin C deficiency	CTV
Zinc deficiency	MIN, BSV, Zinc

Increased Alkaline Phosphatase Continued	
Myositis ossificans	OXCC, OXAA, WO
Neurofibromatosis	OXCC, Hn, #5
Obstructive jaundice	L, Ls, Lb, ACP, GOLD
Osteitis deformans	CAL, Ga, MIN, S
Osteogenic sarcoma	OXAA, OXCC, #5
Osteoporosis	CAL, F+, Ga, Gf, Gb, AZV, MIN
Pancreatic dysfunction	P, Ps
Parasites	VRM-1, 2, 3, 4, WO
Parenchymal jaundice	L, Ls, Lb
Periodontal disease	CAL, WO, GOLD, MIN
Phlebitis	Hcv, OXCC, WO, DSIR
Prostate/uterus problem	Mpc, F+, M+, FPMS
Renal dysfunction	K, Ks, #5, 6
Renal rickets	K, Ks, #6, #5, ACP
Rheumatoid arthritis	ARTA, SENG, #3. Ga, WO
Rickets	AZV, CAL, MIN
Shingles	VIVI, ATAK, DCSU, Hn

Clinical Nutrition:

For Increased ALP

Ga Adrenal
L Liver
Ls Liver Stimulant
LEV Lecithin

PTM Potassium Stabilizer
CAL Calcium Plus
CTV Vitamin C Therapy
BSV Stress B-Vitamin
AZV Multi-Vitamin
D Digestive
#5 Stabilizer
#6 Healer
Magnesium, throughout day
Methionine

For Decreased ALP

PTM Potassium Stabilizer
Ga Adrenal
L Liver
Ls Liver Stimulant

MIN Multi-Mineral
Zinc

Clinical Crossreference:

- **Arthritis** = ↓ Alk. Phos. + ↓ Albumin + ↓ Lymphs + ↓ Copper + ↓ Gamma Globulin + ↓ Neut. + ↓ Platelets + ↑ SGOT + ↑ Uric Acid
- **Brucellosis** = ↑ Alk. Phos. + ↑ WBC + ↑ Lymphs + ↑ Mono + ↑ Neut + ↑ SGPT
- **Congestive Heart Failure** = ↑ Alk. Phos. + ↑ SGOT + ↑ LDH + ↑ (Na^+)

- **Folic Acid Anemia** = ↓ Alk. Phos. + ↑ MCV/MCH
- **Hyperthyroidism** = ↑ Alk. Phos. + ↑ T-3 Uptake
- **Hypothyroidism** = ↓ Alk. Phos. + ↓ T-3 Uptake
- **Liver Dysfunction** = ↑ Alk. Phos. + ↑ SGOT + ↑ GGPT
- **Osteoporosis** = ↑ Alk. Phos. + ↑ Cal. + ↓ Mag.
- **Pancreatic Dysfunction** = ↑ Alk. Phos. + Altered Glucose
- **Parasites** = ↑ Alk. Phos. + ↑ EOS
- **Phlebitis** = ↑ Alk. Phos. + ↑ WBC + ↑ SGOT + ↑ EOS + ↑ Neut. + ↑ Acid Phos. + ↓ Lymphs
- **Possible Hyperadrenals** = ↓ Alk. Phos. + ↓ BUN + ↓ Sodium + ↓ Chlorides
- **Possible Hypoadrenals** = ↑ Alk. Phos. + ↑ BUN + ↑ Potassium
- **Protein Malnutrition** = ↓ Alk. Phos. + ↓ Total Pro.
- **Renal Dysfunction** = ↑ Alk. Phos. + ↑ Creatinine
- **Rheumatoid Arthritis** = ↑ Alk. Phos. + ↑ BUN + ↑ ESR + ↓ HCT + ↓ HGB + ↓ WBC
- **Shingles** = ↑ Alk. Phos. + ↑ BUN + ↑ LDH + ↑ MONO + ↑ Creatinine + ↓ Albumin + ↓ Chol.

Related Tests:

Bilirubin, Cholesterol, GGT, LDH, PHI, SGOT, SGPT, T4, Total Protein, Triglycerides.

Clinical Notes:

- Pregnancy - Alk. Phos. often increases during the third month and remains high until after birth.
- Increased Alk. Phos. results in an alkaline trend in blood pH.
- Decreased Alk. Phos. results in an acid trend in blood pH.
- Biliary tract obstruction usually causes a higher Alk. Phos. than liver disorders.

Practitioner Notes:

- For increased Alk. Phos., magnesium glycinate may need to be used for those with a history of loose stool when magnesium is supplemented. - R.M.
- Rheumatoid Arthritis - rule out food allergies (wheat, corn, milk, beef, nightshade family, chocolate, coffee, alcohol). - J.T.
- Prescription medications can cause elevations and decreases in Alk. Phos. - T.K.
- A decreased Alk. Phos. can be a low adrenal function indicative of impaired phosphate liberation during the utilization of ATP for energy. - J.T.

Other Notes:

ALPHA 1 GLOBULIN

Optimal (Clinical Nutrition) Values 0.2 - 0.3 g/100 ml.

Pathological (Lab) Reference Values: 0.1 - 0.4 g/100 ml.

Alpha 1 Globulin: Indicates the body's catabolic process of breaking down proteins from the muscles and organs to meet its nucleo-protein requirements. Concentrations of Alpha 1 Globulin increase as a result of tissue damage and infections.

Pathological Considerations:

Increased Alpha 1 Globulin	
Carcinomatosis	OXCC, #5, Gt
Catabolic metabolism	PRO
Infections, acute	GOLD, #3
Infections, chronic	#3, ATAK, OXOX
Lupus, systemic eryth	OXAA, OXCC, #5, S
Peptic ulcer	DCSU, AO, #6
Renal dysfunction	K, Ks, #5
Rheumatoid arthritis	ARTA, SENG, #3, WO

Decreased Alpha 1 Globulin	
Gout	K, Ks, Ga, Ls, PTM
Liver dysfunction	L, Ls, #5
Viral hepatitis	L, Ls, VIVI, ATAK

Clinical Nutrition:

For Increased Alpha 1 Globulin

PRO	Nutro-Protein
Gt	Thymus
DSIR	Digestant Internal Regenerator

L Liver
#3 Anti-Infective
P Pancreas

For Decreased Alpha 1 Globulin

L	Liver
Ls	Liver Stimulant

Clinical Crossreference:

- **Catabolic Metabolism** = ↑ Alpha 1 Glob. (See Total Protein)
- **Gout** = ↓ Alpha 1 Glob. + ↑ Uric Acid (See Uric Acid)
- **Hepatitis** = ↑ Alpha 1 Glob. + ↑ SGPT (See SGPT)
- **Infections, Acute and Chronic** = ↑ Alpha 1 Glob. + Alt. WBC (See WBC)
- **Lupus, Systemic Erythematosis** = ↑ Alpha 1 Glob. + ↓ WBC (See WBC)
- **Peptic Ulcer** = ↑ Alpha 1 Glob. + ↑ Gastrin (See Gastrin)

- **Renal Dysfunction** = ↑ Alpha 1 Glob. + ↑ Creatinine (See Creatinine)
- **Rheumatoid Arthritis** = ↑ Alpha 1 Glob. + ↑ Alk. Phos. (See Alk. Phos.)

Related Tests:

Alpha 2 Globulin, Total Globulin, Total Protein

Clinical Notes:

- If protein catabolism is suspected, consider liver or pancreas dysfunction.

Practitioner Notes:

- Alpha 1 Globulin is elevated during fasting and should return to normal shortly after breaking a fast. - J.T.
- Vegetarian athletes often have elevated Alpha 1 Globulin and must focus on Pro-Vita! vegetarian protein meals to meet their bodys' requirements. - J.T.

Other Notes:

ALPHA 2 GLOBULIN

Optimal (Clinical Nutrition) Values 0.6 - 0.9 g/100 ml.

Pathological (Lab) Reference Values: 0.5 - 1.1 g/100 ml.

Alpha 2 Globulin: This fraction determined by protein electrophoresis is indicative of tissue destruction, infections, and inflammatory disease.

Pathological Considerations:

Increased Alpha 2 Globulin	
Carcinoid syndrome	OXCC, #5, Gt
Catabolic metabolism	PRO
Dermatomyositis	#4, ACX, GOLD
Diabetes	P, L, Ls, Gb
Hyperparathyroidism	Gf, Gb
Liver dysfunction	L, Ls, #5
Lupus, systemic eryth	OXCC, #5, OXAA, S
Peptic ulcer	DCSU, AO, #6
Rheumatoid arthritis	ARTA, SENG, #5
Viral hepatitis	L, Ls, VIVI, ATAK

Decreased Alpha 2 Globulin	
Gout	K, Ks, Ga, Ls, PTM
Liver dysfunction	L, Ls, #5
Viral hepatitis	L, Ls, VIVI, ATAK

Clinical Nutrition:

For Increased Alpha 2 Globulin	
PRO	Nutro-Protein
DSIR	Digestant Internal Regenerator
#3	Anti-Infective

L Liver
Ls Liver Stimulant

For Decreased Alpha 2 Globulin	
L	Liver
Ls	Liver Stimulant

Clinical Crossreference:

- **Catabolic Metabolism** = ↑ Alpha 2 Glob. + ↑ Total Protein (See Total Protein)
- **Dermatomyositis** = ↑ Alpha 2 Glob. + ↑ HCT + ↑ ESR + ↑ EOS + ↑ Gamma Glob. + WBC + ↑ LDH + ↓ HGB
- **Diabetes** = ↑ Alpha 2 Glob. + ↑ Glucose (See Glucose)
- **Heart Disease, Ischemic** = ↑ Alpha 2 Glob. + ↑ SGOT + ↑ LDH (See LDH)
- **Hyperparathyroidism** = ↑ Alpha 2 Glob. + ↑ Glob. + ↑ PTH (See PTH)
- **Liver Dysfunction** = ↑ Alpha 2 Glob. + ↑ SGPT (See SGPT)

- **Peptic Ulcer** = ↑ Alpha 2 Glob. + ↑ Gastrin (See Gastrin)
- **Renal Dysfunction** = ↑ Alpha 2 Glob. + ↑ Creat. (See Creat.)
- **Rheumatoid Arthritis** = ↑ Alpha 2 Glob. + ↑ Alk. Phos. (See Alk. Phos.)

Related Tests:

Alpha 1 Globulin, LDH, Total Globulin, Total Protein

Clinical Notes:

- With skin disorders, consider hormonal imbalances (progesterone, testosterone) and liver function. If LDH is elevated with elevated Alpha 2 Globulin, then there is skin and tissue inflammation or destruction.

Practitioner Notes:

- Alpha 2 Globulin elevations are often indicative of the beginning of deeper pathologies specifically Systemic Lupus Erythematosis and Rheumatoid Arthritis. Treat comprehensively. - J.T.

Other Notes:

BASOPHILS (BASO)

Optimal (Clinical Nutrition) Values 0 - 1%

Pathological (Lab) Reference Values: .25 - 2%

Basophils: Are a granulocyte and thus one of the white blood cells comprising up to 2% of the total WBC. The basophil's lysosomes carry powerful enzymes and oxidation agents to help regulate the inflammation process and inhibit the clotting of blood with heparin at the site of inflammation. They also carry enzymes that help with the damaging side effects of inflammation and thus help control histamine and cortisol.

Pathological Considerations:

Increased		Decreased
Anemia, chronic hemolytic	BLDB, MIN, BSV	None known
Blood dyscrasias	OXCC, #5	
Chickenpox	VIVI, ACX	
Chlorosis	OXCC, #5	
Flu	VIVI, ATAK, ACX	
Hypersensitivity, chronic	BSV, MIN	
Hypothyroidism	Gf, #1	
Immune disorders	Gt, #4, S	
Inflammation, systemic	#3, OXOX, Gt	
Leukemia, some	OXCC, #5, S	
Parasites	VRM-1,2,3,4	
Polycythemia	OXAA, #5	
Sinus inflammation	GOLD, #3	
Small pox	VIVI, ATAK	
Spleenectomy, following	S, #6, Gt	

Clinical Nutrition:

For Increased Basophils		For Decreased Basophils
GOLD	**Immune Plus**	
#3	**Anti-Infective**	
Gt	**Thymus**	
CTV	**Vitamin C Therapy**	
MIN	Multi-Mineral	
LEV	Lecithin	
ACP	Vitamin ACP	
Cysteine		

Clinical Crossreference:

- **Chickenpox** = ↑ Baso + ↓ WBC (See WBC)
- **Flu** = ↑ Baso + Alt. WBC (See WBC)
- **Hypothyroidism** = ↑ Baso + ↓ T3 Uptake (See T3 Uptake)

- **Inflammation, Systemic** = ↑ Baso + ↓ Total Protein (See Total Protein)
- **Parasites** = ↑ Baso + ↑ EOS (See EOS)
- **Polycythemia** = ↑ Baso + ↑ HGB (See HGB)

Related Tests:

Lymph, EOS, Mono, Neut., WBC.

Clinical Notes:

- Elevated Baso and EOS is a good indicator of parasitic proliferation. Verify with a comprehensive stool parasite test.

Practitioner Notes:

- A lack of raw food in the diet can cause elevated Baso, general systemic inflammation, and a wearing down of the overall immune function. See *The Pro-Vita Plan For Optimal Nutrition.* - J.T.

Other Notes:

BETA GLOBULIN

Optimal (Clinical Nutrition) Values 0.7 - 1.0 g/100 ml.

Pathological (Lab) Reference Values: 0.6 - 1.2 g/100 ml.

Beta Globulin: The beta fraction of Total Protein can help differentiate abnormalities because it is increased in diabetes, viral hepatitis and rheumatoid arthritis, but unlike the Alpha 1 and 2 Globulins, the Beta Globulin does not increase in response to infections or carcinomatosis.

Pathological Considerations:

Increased Beta Globulin	
Blood lipids, elevated	D, LEV, Ls
Demineralization	MIN, CAL, PTM
Extra-hepatic obstruction	L, Ls, OXCC
Gall bladder dysfunction	Lb, #5, D
Liver dysfunction	L, Ls, #5
Renal dysfunction	K, Ks, #5
Rheumatoid arthritis	ARTA, SENG #3

Decreased Beta Globulin	
Liver dysfunction	L, Ls, #5
Protein digestion dysfunction	D, PRO

Clinical Nutrition:

For Increased Beta Globulin	
Gt	Thymus
L	Liver
Ls	Liver Stimulant

For Decreased Beta Globulin	
L	Liver
Ls	Liver Stimulant
D	Digestive

Clinical Crossreference:

- **Blood Lipids Elevated** = ↑ Beta Glob. + ↑ Trig. (See Trig.)
- **Hepatitis** = ↑ Beta Glob. + ↑ SGPT (See SGPT)
- **Protein Digestion Dysfunction** = ↓ Beta Glob. + ↓ Total Protein (See. Protein, Total)
- **Renal Dysfunction** = ↑ Beta Glob. + ↑ Creat. (See Creat.)

Related Tests:

Alpha 1 Globulin, Alpha 2 Globulin, Gamma Globulin, Total Globulin, Total Protein

Clinical Notes:

- Increased Beta Globulin is associated with demineralization of the body, particularly the bones and soft tissue. It is indicative of the body's inability to utilize minerals.

Practitioner Notes:

- Liver support often helps correct altered Beta Globulin. The liver/immune system connection seems to be exemplified by this fact. - J.T.

Other Notes:

BILIRUBIN, TOTAL

Optimal (Clinical Nutrition) Values: 0.5 - 0.7

Pathological (Lab) Reference Values 0.1 - 1.2
Indirect Bilirubin Lab Values 0.1 - 1.0
Direct Bilirubin Lab Values 0 - 0.2

Total Bilirubin: Bilirubin is the end product of hemoglobin breakdown in the reticuloendothelial system (RES), particularly by the liver Kupffer cells, spleen, and bone marrow. The liver alters bilirubin so it can be excreted via the biliary and renal systems. Total Bilirubin is the sum of Direct Bilirubin (post hepatic conjugated) and Indirect Bilirubin (pre-hepatic unconjugated). When bilirubin is bound to albumin it is indirect, unconjugated, and water insoluble. When it passes through the liver, it is converted to bilirubin diglucuronide and becomes direct, conjugated, and water soluble. Thus, it is best to obtain direct and indirect values to determine if the problem is occurring before or after liver involvement.

Pathological Considerations:

Increased Total Bilirubin

Anemia, hemolytic	BLDB, S, OXAA
Anemia, pernicious	BSV, S
Arsenical intoxication, acute	CLNZ, CTV
Biliary obstruction	Lb, Ls
Catarrhal jaundice	L, Ls, Lb, APHA
Cholecystitis, chronic	Lb, #3
Hepatitis, infectious	L, Ls, #3, #4
Icterus neonatorum	L
Liver injury	L, #6
Mononucleosis	L, Ls, #4, VIVI
Polycythemia vera	S, #5
Thymus dysfunction	Gt

Decreased Total Bilirubin

Aplastic anemia, secondary	BLDB, OXAA
(Usually not clinically significant)	
Barbiturate, salicyalte use	ACX

Increased Direct Bilirubin

Biliary dysfunction	Lb, Ls
Biliary obstruction	
• Calculi	Lb, Flush, KDIR
• Tumor	OXCC, #5, OXAA
Hepatitis, viral	L, Ls, #4
Liver problems	L, Ls

Decreased Direct Bilirubin

No known clinical significance

Increased Indirect Bilirubin

Polycythemia vera	S, #5, OXAA
Spleen dysfunction	S, #5
Hepatitis, viral, later stage	L, Ls, #4
Anemia, several types	BLDB, BSV, MIN, S
Inflammatory conditions	#3, GOLD
Liver dysfunction	L, Ls, OXCC, #5
Biliary dysfunction	Ls, Lb

Decreased Indirect Bilirubin

Spleen dysfunction	S, #3, #5

Clinical Nutrition:

For Increased Total Bilirubin	
L	Liver
Ls	Liver Stimulant
LEV	Lecithin
Gt	Thymus

MIN Multi-Mineral
Methionine
Vitamin B-6
Magnesium
Betaine HCL
Beets

For Decreased Total Bilirubin	
D	Digestive
Lb	Liver Normalizer

S Spleen
BLDB Blood Builder

Clinical Crossreference:

- **Inflammatory Condition** = ↑ Bilirubin (Indirect) + ↑ Basophils
- **Liver/biliary Dysfunction** = ↑ Total Bilirubin + ↑ SGPT + ↑ SGOT
- **Polycythemia Vera** = ↑ Bilirubin (Indirect) + ↑ RBC
- **Spleen Hyperfunction With Depressed Intrinsic Factor** = ↓ Total Bilirubin + ↓ HCT + ↑ Total Iron
- **Splenic Hyperfunction** = ↓ Total Bilirubin, + ↓ HGB + ↓ HCT + ↓ RBC
- **Thymus Dysfunction (Hypo Activity)** = ↑ Total Bilirubin + ↑ HGB + ↑ HCT + ↑ RBC
- **Thymus Hyperfunction** = ↑ Total Bilirubin + ↑ HGB + ↑ HCT + ↑ RBC

Related Tests:

Alkaline Phosphatase, BUN, CBC, Cholesterol, HCT, HGB, LDH, RBC, SGOT, SGPT, Total Iron, Triglycerides.

Clinical Notes:

- Direct Bilirubin is water soluble and is excreted by the kidneys when the liver cells cannot process bilirubin through the biliary ducts to the large intestine. Thus, urinary presence of bilirubin is indicative of liver dysfunction and serves as an excellent early warning for liver toxicity and disease.
- Total Bilirubin concentrations greater than 2.5 mg% often result in jaundice.

Practitioner Notes:

- An increased Total Bilirubin is generally indicative of liver inflammation, gall bladder disease, jaundice, and hemolytic anemia. It also occurs during fasting. - J.T.
- A decreased Total Bilirubin is generally poor digestion of fats due to poor quality or ineffective pH of the bile. - J.T.

- An increased Direct Bilirubin (conjugated) is generally indicative of bile duct blockage or liver disease. - J.T.

* A decreased Direct Bilirubin is generally indicative of Liver/Gall Bladder dysfunction resulting in trouble with fat digestion. - J.T.

- An elevated Indirect Bilirubin (unconjugated) is generally indicative of increased RBC destruction due to hemolytic anemia or spleenic disorder. - J.T.

Other Notes:

BLOOD UREA NITROGEN (BUN)

Optimal (Clinical Nutrition) Values 13 - 18 mg/dl.

Pathological (Lab) Reference Values: 8 - 25 mg/dl.

Blood Urea Nitrogen: Is a waste product formed by the hydrolysis of arginine by arginase in the liver. Urea circulates in the blood and is excreted by the kidneys. Ammonia generated by protein metabolism is converted to urea by a series of enzyme reactions involving ornithine, citrulline, or arginine. If these enzyme systems are impaired, ammonia and urea can increase beyond what the kidneys can process. Urea is also increased by high protein diets and by protein catabolism. Healthy kidneys normally have no difficulty excreting urea because more than 60% of the kidneys must be incapacitated to increase serum urea.

Pathological Considerations:

Increased BUN

RENAL IMPAIRMENT	
Double polycycstic kidney & urinary destruction	K, OXCC, #5
Metallic poisoning	CLNZ, CTV, EZV
Nephritis - acute & chronic	K, GOLD, #3
Prostatic hypertrophy	Mpc, #3, M+
Renal destruction	K, #6
Uremia	K, Ks
Urinary obstruction	KDIR, K
AUGMENTED NITROGEN CATABOLISM	
Carcinoma of stomach	DSIR, OXCC, #5
Dehydration	MIN
Intestinal obstruction	C, APHA, GOLD
Peritonitis, acute general	GOLD, #3, ATAK
Pneumonia	R, GOLD, #4, ATAK, VIVI
Ulcers, peptic & duodenal	DCSU, AO, # 6
OTHER CAUSES	
Addison's disease (high K^+)	Ga, #6, #5
Chelation Therapy (damage)	K, Hcv
Congestive heart failure	H, PTM, EZV, Hcv
Diabetes	L, Ls, Gb, P
GI hemorrhage	AO, DCSU, #6
Gout	K, PTM, Ls, Ga
Liver/Biliary dysfunction	L, Ls, Lb, #5
Loss of tissue	PRO, MIN
Pituitary, anterior dysf.	Gb
Rheumatoid arthritis	ARTA, Ga, WO SENG, #3
Surgical shock	#6, DSIR

Decreased BUN

Acidosis, advanced	Ga, CAL
Acute hepatic insufficiency	L, Ls, #6
Acute liver destruction	L, Ls, OXAA, # 5
Amyloidosis	OXCC, #5
Celiac sprue	DCSU, DSIR, AO
Chronic wasting diseases	PRO, AZV, D, MIN
Liver failure	L, Ls
Malnutrition	PRO, D, MIN
Nephrosis	K, Ks
Pituitary, posterior dysfunction	Gb
Pregnancy	K, L, D

Clinical Nutrition:

For Increased BUN	For Decreased BUN
Gb Pituitary	**Gb Pituitary**
K Kidney	**Ls Liver Stimulant**
L Liver	L Liver
CTV Vitamin C Therapy	#5 Stabilizer
Magnesium	#6 Healer
Asparagus	K Kidney
	Iodine

Clinical Crossreference:

- **Anterior Pituitary Dysfunction And/Or Liver** = ↑ BUN (20-26) (See TSH & SGPT)
- **Blood Iodine, Elevated** = ↑ BUN + ↑ T4 + ↑ T3 + ↑ T7
- **Excess Tissue Fluid, Tendency** = ↓ BUN + ↓ Uric Acid
- **Hyperadrenal, Possible** = ↓ BUN + ↓ Alk. Phos., (K^+) See Potassium
- **Iodine, Depressed** = ↓ BUN + ↑ T4 + ↑ T3 + ↑ T7
- **Poor Protein Utilization** = ↓ BUN + ↑ Protein (See Protein, Total)
- **Posterior Pituitary Dysfunction** = ↓ BUN (8) + Low urine specific gravity (below 1.015)
- **Protein Metabolism Increased (De-Animation)** = ↑ BUN + ↑ Protein

Related Tests:

A/G Ratio, Alkaline Phosphate, BUN/Creatinine Ratio, CPK, Creatinine, Electrolytes, LDH, , Total Protein, Uric Acid.

Clinical Notes:

- Excessively elevated BUN can result in disorientation, mental confusion, and convulsions.
- Toxicity (and over acid liver cells) impairs the biosynthesis of urea causing an increase in ammonia in the body and urine resulting in a high (alkaline) pH. This alkalosis is really a metabolic acidosis.
- Accurate BUN levels are obtained only from a fasting blood test as recently ingested proteins will cause an abnormally high reading.
- BUN changes faster than Creatinine in minor renal problems, thus is a good indicator of kidney dysfunction.
- Decreased BUN is a viable tool for assessing protein deficiencies due to low protein diets and hypochlorhydria.

- Advanced acidosis is often accompanied with painful joints, muscular stiffness on arising, and wandering pains. These same symptoms can also occur in hypochlorhydria.

Warning: A BUN greater than 100 mg/dl is life-threatening.

Practitioner Notes:

- Although inadequate excretion of urea by the kidneys is the most commonly thought of reason for elevated BUN, it is important to consider why the kidneys may be having a difficult time. This leads us to the liver and possibly to a hypertrophied prostate. - J.T.
- A misapplication of the vegetarian diet (low protein, high carbohydrate), can result in an excessively decreased BUN. - J.T.
- An elevated BUN is generally indicative of an underactive anterior pituitary, kidney dysfunction, and dehydration. - J.T.
- A decreased BUN is generally indicative of an overactive anterior pituitary if diet is not influencing it. - J.T.

Other Notes:

BUN/CREATININE RATIO

Optimal (Clinical Nutrition) Values 13 - 15

Pathological (Lab) Reference Values: 12 - 16

BUN/Creat Ratio: Is Blood Urea Nitrogen (BUN) divided by Creatinine (Creat.). The resulting number can provide useful insights to renal (kidney) function and posterior pituitary function. The relationships between these two tissues is established by Vasopressin, the Anti-Diuretic Hormone (ADH) secreted by the posterior pituitary to effect kidney function to retain water.

Pathological Considerations:

Increased BUN/Creat Ratio	
Bleeding, internal	#6, EZV, AO
Blood in GI Tract	AO, DSIR
Burns	#6, AO, DSIR, DCSU
Circulatory failure	Hcv, H
Congestive heart failure	H, PTM, EZV, Hcv
Dehydration	MIN, H_2O
Fever	GOLD, VIVI
High protein diet	Ks, Ls
Pituitary, posterior dysfunction	Gb
Prostatic hypertrophy	Mpc, #3
Renal dysfunction	Ks, K, KDIR, #5
Shock	#6, EE
Tissue trauma	KYRO, #6, BLDB, ACP
Urinary tract obstruction	KDIR, Mpc

Decreased BUN/Creat Ratio (Less than 10)	
ADH, excretion, excessive	Gb
Low protein/high carb. diet	PRO
Pituitary, posterior hypofunction	Gb, #1

Clinical Nutrition:

For Increased BUN/Creat Ratio

Gb Pituitary
BSV Stress B Vitamin

PTM Potassium Stabilizer
MIN Multi-Mineral
Chlorophyll

For Decreased BUN/Creat Ratio

Gb Pituitary
PTM Potassium Stabilizer
BSV Stress B Vitamin

MIN Multi-Mineral

Clinical Crossreference:

- **Posterior Pituitary Dysfunction** = Alt. BUN/Creat. Ratio + Urinary Analysis (Specific gravity pH, osmolality)
- **Renal Dysfunction = BUN/Creat Ratio** = ↑ BUN/Creat Ratio + ↑ Creatinine (See Creatinine)
- **Water In Blood, Decreased & Dietary Proteins, Excessive** = ↑ BUN/Creat Ratio
- **Water In Blood, Increased & Protein Deficiency** = ↓ BUN/Creat Ratio

Related Tests:

A/G Ratio, Alkaline Phosphatase, CPK, Creatinine, Electrolytes, LDH, Total Protein, Uric Acid, Urinalysis.

Clinical Notes:

- Follow *Pro-Vita! Plan for Optimal Nutrition* dietarily.
- Examining BUN/Creat Ratio, A/G Ratio, Cholesterol, Triglycerides, and HDL can provide insights to both protein and fat metabolism.
- Posterior pituitary disorders can cause acidosis as potassium is moved from the inner cell to the extra cellular fluid for excretion via the kidneys.

Practitioner Notes:

- In any posterior pituitary dysfunction, Potassium and Manganese are essential for the body to be able to compensate and correct the abnormal function. - J.T.
- Increased BUN/Creat Ratio is generally indicative of an underactive posterior pituitary, dehydration, or excessive dietary protein. - J.T.
- Decreased BUN/Creat. Ratio is generally indicative of an overactive posterior pituitary, over hydration, or deficient dietary protein. - J.T.

Other Notes:

CALCIUM (Ca ++)

Optimal (Clinical Nutrition) Values 9.7 - 10.1 mg%

Pathological (Lab) Reference Values: 8.5 - 10.5 mg%

Calcium: (Ca^{++}, or Cal.) Is the most abundant mineral in the body. Its roles include repair and maintenance of bones and teeth, transmission of nerve impulses, muscle contraction including heart function, pH balance, and blood clotting. Most of the body's calcium (98%) is stored in the bones as calcium phosphate, and 2% is in the circulation.

Calcium is maintained under tight homeostatic control, thus serum calcium is not an accurate portrayal of the body's calcium situation. If calcium levels fall, calcium is released from the bones. If calcium levels rise, excesses may be stored in the bone or excreted in the urine. The control of calcium in homeostasis is maintained by a complex system including intestinal absorption in the upper part of the small intestine, levels of Vitamin D (ally) and Potassium (antagonist), parathyroid hormone (PTH), and calcitonin (a thyroid hormone). PTH causes calcium to be released from the bone, increases intestinal absorption of calcium, and causes kidney conservation of calcium. Calcitonin causes the kidneys to excrete calcium and assists in re depositing calcium in the bone. Estrogen hormone also assists the introduction of calcium to the bone by increasing osteoblast activity.

Calcium as a nutrient is best in its organic, covalent form as is found in plants rather than in its inorganic, ionic form as found in limestone or dolomite. In the body, calcium exists in two forms: diffusable calcium ions and albumin-bound non-diffusable. Calcium ions are the form that is physiologically active and available for tissue and cellular use. If albumin is low, then the calcium transport system is impaired as is absorption into the body. For every 1 g/dl variation in albumin, calcium levels rise or fall 1.2 mg/dl.

Intestinal absorption of calcium requires an acid medium and Vitamin D. Ultraviolet radiation increases intestinal absorption of calcium, probably through the synthesis of Vitamin D. Some dietary factors can inhibit absorption of calcium including the pasteurization of milk (heat altered, ionically bound calcium) the presence of excessive phosphorous (as in sodas which creates calcium phosphate), and excessive fats (that form insoluble soaps).

Pathological Considerations:

Increased Calcium	
Acromegaly (excess bone growth)	Gb
Alkali Intake, excessive	D, APHA
Carcinoma (metastatic to bone)..	OXAA, OXCC, #5
Hyperparathyroidism	Gf, Gb
Hyperplasia or thyroid tumor....	Gf, OXCC, #5
Hypervitaminosis	Reduce
Multiple myeloma	OXCC, OXAA #5
Neurofibromatosis	OXCC, Hn, #5
Osteoporosis	F+, CAL, MIN
Polycythemia vera	OXAA, BLDB, #5, S

continued

Decreased Calcium	
Acidosis, metabolic	CAL, Ga
Celiac disease	DSIR, DCSU, AO, #6
Diarrhea	PTM, WO
Hemophilia calcipriva	CAL
Hypochlorhydria	D, MIN, Ds
Hypoparathyroidism	Gf, #1
Idiopathic steatorrhea	D, Lb
Malnutrition	PRO, AZV, MIN, D
Necrosis, pancreatic acute	P, OXCC, OXAA
Nephritis severe	K, GOLD, #3

continued

Increased Calcium Continued	
Adrenal cortex hypofunction ...	Ga, #1
Cadmium (heavy metal) toxicity	CLNZ, CTV
Free Radical pathologies	OXCC, #5, CTV
Hypothyroidism	Gf, #1
Ovarian hyperfunction	F+, #6, #5
Pituitary anterior hypofunction	Gb, #1

Decreased Calcium Continued	
Osteomalacia	CAL, MIN AZV
Ovarian hypofunction	F+, #1, Mpr
Pancreatic dysfunction	P, Ps
Pneumonia	R, GOLD, VIVI, #3, 4
Pregnancy	CAL
Protein malnutrition	PRO, D
Renal rickets, dysfunction	K, CAL, Ks
Sprue	DCSU, D, PTM
Tetany (gastric)	D, CAL, AZV
Vitamin D deficiency	AZV, Gf, K

Clinical Nutrition:

For Increased Calcium

D Digestive
ACP Vitamin ACP
MIN Multi-Mineral

CTV Vitamin C Therapy
PRO Nutro-Protein
PTM Potassium Stabilizer
Hydrochloric Acid
Magnesium Orotate
Vitamin A

For Decreased Calcium

D Digestive
Ps Pancreas Stabilizer
CAL Calcium Plus

P Pancreas
Gf Thyroid *Note: Gf Thyroid formula also supports the parathyroid glands.*
Vitamin D

Clinical Crossreference:

- **Adrenal Hyperfunction** = ↑ Calcium + ↑ Potassium (See Potassium)
- **Cadmium (Heavy Metal) Toxicity** = ↑ Calcium + ↓ Phos. + ↓ Urinary Phosphorus + ↓ MCV
- **Gall Bladder Emulsification, Poor** = ↓ Calcium + ↑ Phosphorus
- **Gastric Intrinsic Problem, Possible** = ↑ Calcium + ↓ Phosphorus
- **Hydrochloric Acid Deficiency Or Hypervitaminosis** = ↑ Calcium + ↑ Phosphorus
- **Hypo/Hyper Parathyroidism** = See PTH
- **Hypothyroidism** = ↑ Calcium + ↓ T3 Uptake
- **Intestinal Absorption of Fat, Poor** = ↓ Calcium + ↓ Bilirubin + ↓ Phosphorus
- **Osteoporosis** = ↓ Calcium + ↑ Alk. Phos. (See Alk. Phos.)
- **Pancreas Dysfunction** = ↓ Calcium + Alt. Glucose (See Glucose)
- **Pancreatic Enzyme Deficiency** = ↓ Calcium + ↓ Triglycerides + ↑ LDH
- **Protein Assimilation, Poor** = ↓ Calcium + ↓ Protein

- **Vitamin D Insufficiency** = ↓ Calcium + ↓ Phosphorus + ↑ Alkaline Phosphatase

Related Tests:

Alkaline Phosphatase, Calcintonin, Calcium/Albumin Ratio, CBC, Growth Hormone, Parathyroid Hormone, Phosphorus, Pituitary, Total Protein, Vitamin D.

Clinical Notes:

- Serum Calcium, in conjunction with phosphorus and PTH, provides excellent insight to parathyroid function.
- Stress depletes calcium.
- During pregnancy, compare calcium and phosphorus, figure the ratio to monitor calcium levels.
- Diets with excessive red meat deplete calcium and contribute to osteoporosis.

Practitioner Notes:

- When sodium is low, the body will use calcium in the bicarbonate buffer system to maintain blood pH in the presence of dietary or metabolic acids. A sodium deficiency may precede excessive calcium loss. - J.T.
- For more information on calcium and bone loss, read "Osteoporosis; the Preventable Disease" and "The Menopause Myth". (See Catalog)
- An elevated Calcium is generally indicative of hyperparathyroidism, bone demineralization, blood clotting problems and cancer. - J.T.
- An increased Calcium is generally indicative of dietary insufficiency, thyroid dysfunction (increased calcitonin secretion) and disorders of fat metabolism. - J.T.

Other Notes:

CARBON DIOXIDE (CO_2)

Optimal (Clinical Nutrition) Values 26 - 28 mEq./l.

Pathological (Lab) Reference Values: 22 - 32 mEq./l.

Carbon Dioxide: (CO_2) Is the primary bicarbonate buffering agent (alkaline reserve) for neutralization of metabolic and dietary acids, a function that is regulated by the kidneys. 95% of the total CO_2 is bicarbonate (HCO_3). The remaining 5% is dissolved CO_2 gas and carbonic acid (H_2CO_3) and is regulated by the lungs. This test measures the effectiveness of gas exchange in the lungs, but primarily provides insights to the pH (acid/alkaline) balance when substantiated by urine and salivary pH analysis.

Pathological Considerations:

Increased Carbon Dioxide

ALKALOSIS: Above 32 mEq/l + low chlor.

Aldosteronism	Ga, PTM, K
Alkali, excessive therapy	PRO APHA
Emphysema	R, # 3, 4, 5, ATAK
Fevers	GOLD, ATAK
Hypercorticoadrenalism	Ga, Gb, PTM
Intestinal alkalosis, congenital	APHA, BIF, C
Oxygen therapy, side effect	PRO, APHA
Pyloric obstruction	DCSU , DSIR
Respiratory impairment	R, Hcv
Tetany	AZV, Gf, CAL, MIN
Typhus fever	GOLD, #3, PTM
Vomiting, acute	WO
Mercury toxicity	CLNZ, CTV

Decreased Carbon Dioxide

ACIDOSIS: Mild acidosis: 18 - 24 mEq/l
Moderate acidosis: 14 - 18 mEq/l
Severe acidosis: less than 14 mEql

Aspirin, (salicyalte)	DCSU
Diabetes	P, Ls, L, Gb
Dehydration	K, Ks, AO
Eclampsia	N3, Nc
Renal dysfunction	K, Ks
Toxic conditions	ACX, CLNZ, SENG CTV

Clinical Nutrition:

For Increased CO_2

R Lung
ACX Vitamin Detox
Ga Adrenal

Correct pH (APHA pH Control)

For Decreased CO_2

R Lung
ACX Vitamin Detox
Ga Adrenal

K Kidney
MIN Multi-Mineral
Correct pH

Clinical Crossreference:

- **Acidosis** = ↓ (CO_2) + ↓ CAL + ↑ Chlor. + ↑ (K^+)
- **Alkalosis** = ↑ (CO_2) + ↓ CAL + ↓ Chlor. + ↓ (K^+) +↓ BUN
- **Diabetes** = ↓ (CO_2) + ↑ Glucose + ↑ Trig. + ↑ LDH
- **Hypercorticoadrenalism** = ↑ (CO_2) + ↓ (K^+) + ↑ (Na^+) + ↑ Chlor. + ↓ Renin + ↑ Cortisol

- **Respiratory Distress** = ↑ Total Protein (See Protein, Total)

Related Tests:

Alkaline Phosphate, Bilirubin, CO_2, Cortisol, Creatinine, Electrolytes, Glycohemoglobin, GGTP, SGOT, Total Protein, Triglycerides.

Clinical Notes:

- Follow *Pro-Vita Plan! For Optimal Nutrition* dietarily. (See Catalog)

- In acidosis states of diabetes, the excessive ketoacids delete the bicarbonate buffer resulting in a low CO_2.

Warning:

- A CO_2 value less than 6.1 is a medical emergency. The condition is critical metabolic acidosis.

Practitioner Notes:

- An increased CO_2 is generally indicative of respiratory acidosis, metabolic alkalosis, and overactive adrenals. - J.T.

- A decreased CO_2 is generally indicative of respiratory alkalosis, metabolic acidosis, and adrenal fatigue. - J.T.

Other Notes:

CHLORIDE (CL^-)

Optimal (Clinical Nutrition) Values: 100 - 105 mEq./l.

Pathological (Lab) Reference Values 95 - 109 mEq./l.

Chloride: (CL^-) Is an electrolyte (anion) element involved in fluid osmality and pH (acid/alkaline balance) in the body. The majority of chloride levels in the body come from salt, or hydrochloric acids. Chlorides, along with sodium, potassium, and CO_2, form the basis of pH (the acid/alkaline dynamic.) Chloride helps regulate the cellular osmotic pressure. This test is conducted to reveal kidney, adrenal, electrolyte, and parathyroid disorders.

Pathological Considerations:

Increased Chloride	
Adrenal cortex hyperfunction	Ga, Gb, PTM
Anemia	BLDB, MIN, BSV, S, Lb
Bowel dysfunction	C
Cardiac decompensation	Hcv, H
CO_2 deficient (acidosis)	Ga
Cushing's syndrome	Gb, KDIR, P, OXCC, #5
Dehydration	MIN, AO
Eclampsia	N3, Nc
Hyperventilation, low CO_2	R, Ga
Hypoproteinemia	PRO, D, Ds
Nephritis	K, #3, GOLD
Nephroses	K, Ks, KDIR
Prostatic, obstruction	M+, W/ WO, Mpc, KDIR
Salicylate Poisoning	Ls, ACX, CTV, L
Serum sickness	BLDB, Lb, D

Decreased Chloride	
Addison's disease	Ga, #5
Anaphylactic shock	Ga, ACX
Bladder dysfunction	K
Burns, Extensive	DCSU, #6, AO, WO
CO_2 excess (alkalosis)	APHA, R
Diabetic acidosis	P, L, Ls, Gb, CAL
Diarrhea	PTM
Eclampsia (with vomiting)	Nc, N3
Emphysema	R, #3, 4, 5, ATAK
Ether anesthesia	ACX
Excessive vomiting	WO
Fevers--acute infections	GOLD, #3, VIVI, ATAK
Generalized edema	Ks, KDIR, K, DSIR
Heat cramps	MIN, PTM
Hypercorticoadrenalism	Ga, Gb, PTM
Intestinal alkalosis congenital	APHA, BIF, C
Intestinal obstruction	C, GOLD
Mercury poisoning	CLNZ, CTV
Nephritis, advanced	K, #3, GOLD
Perspiration, excessive	MIN, PTM
Pneumonia	R, #3, 4, ATAK
Pyloric spasm	D, #6, MIN, DCSU, DSIR
Tetany (bicarbonate)	AZV, Gf, CAL, MIN
Typhus fever	GOLD, #3, PTM
Ulcerative colitis	DCSU, DSIR, WO #6, BIF, BSV, GOLD
Uremia	K, Ks, ACX

Clinical Nutrition:

For Increased Chloride	For Decreased Chloride
Ks Kidney Stabilizer	Ga Adrenal
K Kidney	K Kidney
D Digestive	MIN Multi-Mineral
C Colon	LEV Lecithin
Gb Pituitary	APHA pH Control
Pyridoxine	BSV Stress B-Vitamin
	Magnesium
	Chlorophyll

Clinical Crossreference:

- **Adrenal Cortex Hypofunction** = ↓ Chloride + ↑ (K^+) + ↑ Renin + ↓ (Na^+) + ↓ Cortisol + ↓ Aldesterone + ↓ (CO_2)
- **Adrenal Cortex Hyperfunction** = ↑ Chloride + ↓ (K^+) + ↑ (Na^+) + ↑ Cortisol + ↑ Aldosterone + ↑ (CO_2) + ↓ Renin
- **CO2 Deficient** = ↑ Chloride + ↓ (CO_2) + ↓ Cal. + ↑ (K^+)
- **CO2 Excess** = ↓ Chloride + ↑ (CO_2)+ ↓ Cal. + ↓ (K^+) + ↑ BUN
- **Pyloric Spasm** = ↓ Chlorides + ↓ (K^+) + ↓ (Na^+) + ↑ Gastrin
- **Renal Dysfunction** = ↑ Chloride + ↑ Creatinine + ↑ Acid Phos. + ↓ (CO_2) + ↓ Cal.
- **Respiratory Distress** = ↓ Chlorides + ↑ Total Protein + ↑ BUN + ↑ Uric Acid + ↑ (K^+) + ↑ Triglycerides + ↓ Bilirubin + ↓ Cortisol (See Total Protein)
- **Salicylate Poisoning (Excessive Use Of Aspirin)** = ↑ Chlorides + ↓ RBC + Anemic Trend
- **Water Crossing Cell Membranes (Too Little, Edema)** = ↓ Chlorides + ↓ Albumin
- **Water Crossing Cell Membranes (Too Much)** = ↑ Chlorides

Related Tests:

Alkaline Phosphatase, BUN, CBC, Cholesterol, CO_2, Creatinine, Glucose, HCT, HGB, LDH, Potassium, SGOT, SGPT, Total Iron, Total Protein, Triglycerides.

Clinical Notes:

- Chloride, sodium, and potassium ions are present on both sides of the cell plasma membrane. The electrical potentials of these ions from the field for the exchange of nutrients and glucose from the extra cellular fluids to the inner cell environment, and the excretion of metabolic wastes from the inner cell to the lymph for removal or reorganization. Chloride ions are primarily extra cellular.

- Chloride provides insights to adrenal medula, kidney, bladder, and bowel function regarding fluid and gas exchange across cell membranes.
- Chlorides are usually inverse to CO_2, so high chlorides are common in acidosis, and low chlorides are common with alkalosis.
- In metabolic acidosis, chlorides rise as bicarbonate levels drop.
- When the adrenal hormone Aldosterone initiates an increase in the reabsorption of sodium (Na^+), chlorides also increase to maintain ionic balance.
- *See Pro-Vita! Plan For Optimal Nutrition* for chapter on pH, how to measure. (See Catalog)

Warning:

- Serum chloride below 70 or above 120 indicates an emergency electrolytic imbalance or cellular osmotic pressure imbalance.

Practitioner Notes:

- Low chloride with/without low sodium levels can mean low salt intake. For competition athletes and persons doing more than 60 minutes of hard cardiovascular exercise every other day or more, trace minerals may be the best way to restore chloride. - R.M.
- An increased chloride is generally indicative of an overactive posterior pituitary, respiratory alkalosis, and dehydration. - J.T.
- A decreased chloride is generally indicative of adrenal, kidney, and respiratory inability to regulate pH. - J.T.

Other Notes:

CHOLESTEROL

Optimal (Clinical Nutrition) Values 170 - 200 mg/dl.

Pathological (Lab) Reference Values: 120 - 250 mg/dl.

Cholesterol: Is a steroid fatty (lipid) substance found in all body cells and plasma. It is produced primarily by the liver but also derived by diet. Cholesterol is a cellular body builder at its optimal values. At the pathological values it can be disastrous, leading to heart disease, stroke, atherosclerosis and arteriosclerosis.

As a fatty substance, cholesterol does not dissolve in water and must be encountered around the body with the help of lipoproteins. There are several types of lipoproteins that can escort cholesterol: low density lipoprotein (LDH), high density lipoprotein (HDL), and very low density lipoprotein (VLDL). Basically, LDL cholesterol is the form that sticks to artery walls and causes heart attacks, and HDL cholesterol is able to protect against heart attacks by removing excessive cholesterol from the artery walls and circulating it back to the liver for further processing. Thus, cholesterol is "good" or "bad" according to its form and quantity.

Cholesterol and other lipids are controlled by the liver along with several other organ systems including the thyroid, adrenals, pituitary, pancreas, micelles, and kidney; as well as by diet and fiber in the diet. If thyroid function is low, the liver is sluggish. If the liver is sluggish, it may not function to esterize cholesterol and also not enough bile is formed to allow proper excretion of cholesterol. A reason for a sluggish thyroid is often a low thyroid stimulating hormone (TSH) output from the pituitary. Insulin and glucogen from the pancreas influence cholesterol levels. During stress, cholesterol elevates due to the response of the kidneys, the pancreas (glucagon) and adrenals (catlcholamine). The micelles are involved with the absorption of cholesterol into the bloodstream. Thus, there are many factors and tissues that have a bearing on cholesterol.

Most people in the USA are aware of the dangers of elevated LDL cholesterol which include atherosclerosis and coronary artery disease. Few are informed about the important role cholesterol plays in overall good health. Cholesterol is important for cell wall structure, cellular immunity, steroid production, membrane strength, formation of bile acids, and nerve insulation. Decreased cholesterol levels must be viewed as a health concern, particularly since they frequently accompany auto-immune diseases.

Pathological Considerations:

Increased Cholesterol	
Arteriosclerosis	Hcv, D (w/o food)
Atherosclerosis	D (w/o food), Hcv, CTV, LEV, FLX
Cardiac dysfunction	Hcv, H
Celiac disease	D
Coronary artery disease	Hcv, FLX
Diabetes mellitus	P, L, Ls, Gb
Eclampsia	Nc, N3
Glomerulonephritis, chronic	K, Ks, KDIR
Hemophilia	AZV
Hypothyroidism	Gf, #1
Lipemia	D (w/o food)
Liver disease	L, LS
Lukemia	S, OXCC, #5, BLDB
Lupus, systemic erthimatosis	OXCC, S, #3, VIVI, ATAK
Malingancy	OXCC, #5

Decreased Cholesterol	
Anemia (pernicious)	BLDB, MIN, BSV
Auto-immune diseases	OXCC, Gt, #5
Cachexia	AZV, MIN, PRO
Cardiac dysfunction	H, HCV
Endocrine dysfunction	Gb, Gf, Ga
Epilepsy	B, Ls, L, #4
Free-radical pathologies	CTV, EZV, CLNZ
Gaucher's disease	L, Ls, S, SENG
Hemolytic Jaundice	L, Ls, Lb
Hepatic insufficiency	L, Ls
Hepatitis	L, GOLD, VIVI
Hypothyroidism	Gf, Gb
Inanition	AZV, MIN, PRO
Infection, acute	GOLD, #3, VIVI
Infections, acute	GOLD, ATAK, #3
Intestinal obstruction	C

Increased Cholesterol Continued	
Multiple sclerosis	FLX, Hn, OXCC, #5, CAL, EZV
Nephrosis	K, Ks
Obstructive jaundice	L, Ls, Lb
Pancreas dysfunction	P, Ps
Pregnancy	L, Ls, Hcv
Prostate, benign hypertrophy	Mpc, Mpr, #3
Renal dysfunction	K, Ks
Xanthomatosis	D (W/O foo), LEV

Decreased Cholesterol Continued	
Libido, low	M+, F+
Liver/gall bladder dysfunction	L, Ls, Lb
Mononucleosis	L, Ls, #4, VIVI
Polycythemia	BLDB, OXAA, #5
Protein malnutrition	PRO, D
Shingles	VIVI, ATAK, Hn, DCSU
Stress, cracks under	Hn, Ga, MIN, BSV
Uremia	K, Ks

Clinical Nutrition:

For Increased Cholesterol

Ls Liver Stabilizer
Gf Thyroid
PTM Potassium Stabilizer
LEV Lecithin
Hcv Cardiovascular
Ps Pancreas Stabilizer
FLX Flax-Seed Oil
EZV Vitamin E 200
BSV Stress B-Vitamin
K Kidney
Methinonine
Magnesium
Pro-Vita! Plan
Vitamin B-6
To Elevate HDL: EZV Vitamin E 200
Chromium
GLA

For Decreased Cholesterol

LEV Lecithin
BSV Stress B-Vitamin
Gt Thymus
#4 Corrector
Methionine

Clinical Crossreference:

- **Multiple Sclerosis** = ↑ Cholesterol + ↑ IgE + ↑ GGTP + ↑ Alpha 1 & 2 + ↑ Albumin + ↑ Beta Gamma Globulin + ↓ Phospholipids + ↓ Vit. B-12 + ↓ Lymphs
- **Mental Retardation** = ↓ Cholesterol + ↑ Glutamic Acid
- **Diabetes** = ↑ Cholesterol + ↑ Glucose + ↑ Triglycerides + ↑ LDH + ↑ SGOT
- **Protein Malnutrition** = ↓ Cholesterol + ↓ Total Protein (See Total Protein)
- **Gout** = ↑ Cholesterol + ↑ Uric Acid (See Uric Acid)
- **Arteriosclerosis** = ↑ Cholesterol + ↑ BUN + ↑ CO_2 + ↑ LDL (VLDL) + ↑ Copper + ↑ Uric Acid + ↑ Creatinine + ↑ Cholesterol + ↑ Triglycerides + ↓ HDL
- **Liver/Biliary Dysfunction** = ↑ Cholesterol + ↑ SGPT + ↑ GGTP (See SGPT)
- **Pancreatic Dysfunction** = ↑ Cholesterol + ↑ Glucose (See Glucose)

- **Renal Dysfunctioon** = ↑ Cholesterol + ↑ Creatinine (See Creatinine)
- **Endocrine Dysfunction** = ↑ Cholesterol + ↓ T3 Uptake (See T3 Uptake)
- **Cardiac Dysfunction** = ↑ Cholesterol + ↑ SGOT (See SGOT)
- **Lupus** = ↑ Cholesterol + ↓ WBC (See WBC)
- **Shingles** = ↓ Cholesterol + ↑ Alk. Phos (See Alk. Phos.)
- **Prostate, Benign Hypertrophy** = ↑ Cholesterol + ↑ Creatinine (See Creatinine)
- **Hepatitis** = ↓ Cholesterol + ↑ SGPT (See SGPT)
- **Mononucleosis** = ↓ Cholesterol + ↑ SGPT (See SGPT)

Related Tests:

Alkaline Phosphatase, BUN, SGOT, SGPT, T3, T4, T7, Total Protein, Triglycerides, TSH.

Clinical Notes:

- *Your Liver...Your Lifeline* outlines the gall bladder flush program. (See Catalog).
- HDL is primarily a phospholipid, the only known carrier of cholesterol-plaque from the arteries to the liver.
- Bile is the carrier of excessive cholesterol out of the body.
- HDL cholesterol can be converted to other lipo-proteins by an enzyme, lecithin-cholesterol acytranferase (LCAT).
- *The Pro-Vita! Plan for Optimal Nutrition* discusses the appropriate diet.(See Catalog).

Practitioner Notes:

- Increased cholesterol is generally indicative of a high fat diet, low adrenal function, low thyroid function and pancreas dysfunction. - J.T.
- Decreased cholesterol is generally indicative of poor digestion of fats, hormonal imbalance and liver dysfunction. - J.T.

Other Notes:

CREATININE

Optimal (Clinical Nutrition) Values: 0.8- 1.0 mg/dl.

Pathological (Lab) Reference Values:
Men: 0.7 - 1.6 mg/dl.
Women: 0.6 - 1.2 mg/dl.

Creatinine: Is the end result of creatine phosphate, a chemical in our bodies used in the energy metabolism of muscle contraction. Like Blood Urea Nitrogen, Creatinine is filtered through the kidneys and is a method to monitor the progress of kidney diseases or ascertain general kidney health. In renal dysfunctions the creatinine and BUN levels in serum approximate each other. In sub-acute renal dysfunctions, the BUN elevates at a faster rate.

Pathological Considerations:

Increased Creatinine	
Atrophy & Dystrophy (Muscular)	KYRO, Hn, #5, PTM, MIN
Congestive heart failure	H
Diabetes, uncontrolled	L, Ls, P, Gb, Ps
Early nephritis (2-4 mg.)	K, GOLD
Gout	K, Ks, PTM, Ga
Intestinal obstruction	C, AO
Prostate, benign hypertrophy	Mpc, Mpr, M+
Prostatic obstruction	Mpc, KDIR, GOLD, M+, WO
Renal dysfunction	K, #6
Severe nephritis (4-35 mg.)	K, #3, GOLD
Starvation	PRO, AZV, MIN
Urinary obstruction	KDIR, K

Decreased Creatinine	
Amyotonia congenita	KYRO, LEV
Growth, children	AZV, MIN
Muscle atrophy/dystrophy	KYRO, PRO, ACP #6, MIN
Pregnancy	K, PTM

(below .7 not clinically significant)

Clinical Nutrition:

For Increased Creatinine

CTV Vitamin C Therapy
FLX Flax Seed Oil

Kidneys:
- K Kidney
- Ks Kidney Stabilizer
- ACP Vitamin ACP

Muscle:
- KYRO Tissue Strengthener
- EZV Vitamin E 200
- MIN Multi-Mineral
- Selenium
- Di-methyl Glycine

Prostate
- Mpc Prostata Candida
- Mpr Prostata/Ovatum
- M+ Male Endocrine
- Zinc

For Decreased Creatinine

KYRO Tissue Strengthener
LEV Lecithin

MIN Multi-Mineral
ACP Vitamin ACP
EZV Vitamin E 200
PRO Nutro-Protein
PTM Potassium Stabilizer

Clinical Crossreference:

- **Congestive Heart Failure** = ↑ Creat. + ↑ SGOT + ↑ LDH
- **Diabetes** = ↑ Creat. + ↑ Trig. + ↑ BUN + ↑ Chol. + ↑ U. A. + ↑ Glucose + ↑ Acid Phosphatase + ↑ LDH + ↑ SGOT
- **Gout** = ↑ Creat. + ↑ Uric Acid
- **Muscle Atrophy** = ↓ Creat. + ↑ CPK
- **Prostate Hypertrophy, Benign** = ↑ Creat. + ↑ Acid Phos. + ↑ MONO + ↑ Progosterone + ↑ BUN + ↑ Uric Acid + ↑ Testosterone
- **Renal Dysfunction** = ↑ Creat. + ↑ Acid Phosphotase + ↑ Chloride + ↓ CO_2 + ↓ Calcium + ↑ Phosphorus + ↓ Albumin + ↓ HCT/HGB + ↑ BUN +↑ Uric Acid + ↑ LDH + ↑ SGOT

Related Tests:

Aldolase, BUN Urinalysis, Cholinesterase, T4, Uric Acid.

Clinical Notes:

- A person with a known kidney dysfunction may have a normal Creatinine value in which case Creatinine cannot be used to evaluate function of progress.
- Creatinine differs from BUN in that it is not effected by dietary protein, gender, or protein catabolism.
- High animal flesh diets can elevate Creatinine.

Warning: A Creatinine elevated above 10 mg/dl. indicates a medical emergency.

Practitioner Notes:

- If BUN/Creat. Ratio is less than 10, increase dietary protein. If there already is adequate dietary protein, check for malabsorption. - R.M.
- People taking mega doses of Vitamin C can have increased Creatinine levels not indicative of kidney dysfunction. - J.T.
- Increased Creatinine is generally indicative of impaired kidney function or excessive muscle breakdown. - J.T.
- Decreased Creatinine is generally overactive kidney function. - J.T.

Other Notes:

EOSINOPHILS (EOS)

Optimal (Clinical Nutrition) Values 0 - 2%

Pathological (Lab) Reference Values: 0 - 7%

Eosinophils: Are one of six primary leukocytes (white blood cells) dedicated to fighting infections. Eosinophils can engulf pathogens (phagocytosis) and contain several enzymes involved in the deactivation of mediators of the inflamation response. One of these specialized enzymes is Histaminase which reduces cellular induration resultant from the histamine reaction. Since Eosinophils play a role in moderating certain inflammatory responses, they are increased when such situations exist. The primary situations which cause activation of eosinophil production are allergies and intestinal parasites. Eosinophils can also be increased in skin diseases, respiratory disorders, some leukemias, some cancers, autoimmune diseases, adrenal insufficiency, and following radiation therapy. Eosinophils are formed in the bone marrow and migrate to the spleen where they mature and are viable for 8 - 12 days. Normally they make 1% - 3% of the white blood cells in the body.

Pathological Considerations:

Increased Eosinophils

Allergic Conditions

Angio-neurotic edema	ACX, Ga, KDIR
Bronchial Asthma	R, Ga, *Zinc*
Food allergy	D, BIF,. DSIR, L, Ls
Hay Fever	ACX, Ga, Gt
Urticaria	ACX, Ga

Blood Dyscrasias

Hodgkin's Diease	OXCC, OXAA, #5, S, Gt
Inflamation of Arteries	ACX, #3, HCV, GOLD
Pernicious Anemia	BSV, BLDB, MIN

Infections

Chorea	#3, ATAK, OXOX
Gonorrhea, Chronic	ATAK, #4, VIVI
Scarlet Fever	GOLD, VIVI, S

Miscellaneous

Adrenal insufficiency	Ga
Free-radical pathologies	OXCC, #5, CTV
Loeffler's Syndrome	GOLD, VIVI
Molluscum contagiosum	VIVI, TR, WO
Periarteritis nodosa	Hcv, CTV

Parasitic Diseases

Echinococcal Disease	L, VRM-4
Infestation with Liver Fluke	VRM-4, WO
Schistosomiasis	VRM-2, VRM-4
Some Intestinal Parasites	VRM-1, VRM-3
Trichinosis	VRM-2, WO

continued...

Decrease Eosinophils

No known clinical significance

ACTH injections	Ga
Post surgery	#6, AZV, MIN
Post radiation therapy	ACX, Gt, AZV

Increased Eosinophils Continued...	
Skin Diseases	
Dermatitis Herpetiformis	VIVI, DSCU
Adrenal cortex hypofunction	Ga, #1
Dermatomyositis	ACP, KYRO, #6
Hyperthyroidism	Gf, #5, Gb
Pemphigus	#3, REV, XL
Phlebitis	Hcv, OXCC, WO
Pituitary, anterior hypofunction .	Gb
Polycythemia	OXAA, #5
Rheumatoid Arthritis	ARTA, #3, SENG
Tumors, ovary, bone, serous	OXCC, #5, OXAA

Clinical Nutrition:

For Increased Eosinophils

CTV Vitamin C Therapy
CAL Calcium Plus
S Spleen
Vitamin D
Ps Pancreas Stimulant
VRM-1,2,3,4
Pantothenic Acid

For Decreased Eosinophils

No therapy indicated

Clinical Crossreference:

- **Dermatomyositis** = ↑ EOS + ↑ Alpha 2 Globulin + ↑ ESR + ↑ LDH + ↑ Gamma Globulin + ↑ WBC + ↓ HGB
- **Environment Allergies** = ↑ EOS + ↑ I_gE
- **Food Allergies** = ↑ EOS + ↑ I_gE
- **Hyperthyroidism** = ↑ EOS + ↑ T3 Uptake (See T3 Uptake)
- **Parasites** = ↑ EOS + ↑ Occult Blood (Stool) + ↑ Total Globulin + ↑ I_gE + ↓ Serum Iron + ↓ MCH + ↓ MCHC + ↓ MCV + ↓ HGB + ↓ HCT + ↓ RBC
- **Phlebitis** = ↑ EOS + ↓ Alk. Phos.
- **Rheumatoid Arthritis** = + ↑ EOS + ↑ Alk. Phos (See Alk. Phos.)

Related Tests:

Baso, Lymphs, Monos, Neut, WBC.

Clinical Notes:

- In prolonged infections, eosinophils can decrease to zero, and reappear when the body recovers.

Practitioner Notes:

• By following the Pro-Vita! Plan dietarily, elevated EOS can normalize without therapeutic treatment if the elevation is based on misuse of animal protein and excessive dairy intake - J.T.

Other Notes:

ERYTHROCYTE SEDIMENTATION RATE (ESR)

Optimal (Clinical Nutrition) Values
Male: 0 - 5 mm/hr.
Female: 0 - 10 mm/hr.

Pathological (Lab) Reference Values:
Male: 0 - 10 mm/hr.
Female: 0 - 20 mm/hr.

Erythrocyte Sedimentation (ESR): Also called "Sed Rate" is an indicator if there is inflammation or tissue destruction. It is not for any specific disease, but serves as notification of a problem and can be used to monitor improvement or degeneration. "Erythrocyte" refers to the red blood cell. "Sedimentation rate" refers to the clumping together of cells. Fibrinogen, a liver-derived glycoprotein and precursor to fibrin (blood clotting factor) increases in the plasma when inflammation and tissue destruction occur, as well as in pregnancy and auto immune disorders. The increased plasma fibrinogen causes an increased Sed Rate. An increase in albumin will decrease fibrinogen and the sed rate, thus if the liver is unable to synthesize albumin effectively, the Sed Rate will rise.

Pathological Considerations:

Increased ESR	
Dermatomyositis	#4, ACX, GOLD
Free Radical pathologies	OXCC, OXAA, CTV
Gout	K, Ks, Ga, Ls, PTM
Heart dysfunction	H, Hcv, #5
Hyperparathyroidism	Gf, Gb
Hepatitis	L, Ls, #4, GOLD
Inflammatory states	#3, OXOX, GOLD
Liver dysfunction	L, Ls, #5
Mumps	VIVI, ACX
Parasitic conditions	VRM-1,-2,-3,-4
Thyroid dysfunction	Gf, #5

Decreased ESR
No known significance (Zero is optimal)

Clinical Nutrition:

For Increased ESR	
OXCC	**Cell Cleanser**
#5	**Stabilizer**
L	**Liver**
Ls	**Liver Stimulant**
#3	Anti-Infective
#4	Corrector

For Decreased ESR

Clinical Crossreference:

- **Dermatomyositis** = ↑ ESR + ↑ Alpha 2 Glob. (See Alpha 2 Glob.)
- **Gout** = ↑ ESR + ↑ Uric Acid (See Uric Acid)
- **Heart Dysfunction** = ↑ ESR + ↑ SGOT (See SGOT)
- **Hepatitis** = ↑ ESR + ↑ SGPT (See SGPT)
- **Inflammatory Conditions** = ↑ ESR + Alt. WBC (See WBC)
- **Influenza** = ↑ ESR + Alt. WBC (See WBC)
- **Hyperparathyroidism** = ↑ ESR + ↑ PTH (See PTH)
- **Liver Dysfunction** = ↑ ESR + ↑ SGPT (see SGPT)
- **Mumps** = ↑ ESR + ↑ WBC (See WBC)
- **Parasitic Conditions** = ↑ ESR + ↑ EOS (See EOS)
- **Rheumatoid Arthritis** = ↑ ESR + ↑ Alk. Phos. (See Alk. Phos.)
- **Thyroid Dysfunction** = ↑ ESR + Alt. T-3 Uptake (See T-3 Uptake)

Related Tests:

Alk. Phos., SGPT, WBC

Clinical Notes:

- The reason females are allowed a higher ESR than men is to account for the menstrual cycle.
- To verify liver involvement in an elevated ESR, check liver function tests.

Practitioner Notes:

- Use ESR to monitor nutritional and therapeutic alleviation of rheumatoid arthritis. - J.T.

Other Notes:

FOLLICLE STIMULATING HORMONE (FSH)

Optimal (Clinical Nutrition) Values 4 - 20 mIU/ml

Pathological (Lab) Reference Values:
Male 4 - 25 mIU/ml
Female 4 - 30 mIU/ml

Follicle Stimulating Hormone: Is a glycopeptide hormone secreted by the anterior pituitary. Along with the Luetinizing hormone, FSH is responsible to stimulate the function of the ovaries or the testes. The secretion of FSH is controlled by the hypothalamus which receives input regarding the function of the gonads via the bloodstream.

Pathological Considerations:

Increased FSH	
Hot flashes	Fpms, Gf
Menopause	F+, Fpms, Gb

Decreased FSH	
Pituitary, anterior hypofunction	Gb, #1

Clinical Nutrition:

For Increased FSH	
Fpms	Female PMS
Gb	Pituitary
Gf	Thymus
F+	Female Plus

For Decreased FSH	
Gb	Pituitary
#1	Activator

Clinical Crossreference:

- **Pituitary, Anterior Hypofunction** = ↓ FSH + ↓ TSH (See TSH)

Related Tests:

Luetinizing Hormone, TSH

Clinical Notes:

- Confirm anterior pituitary hypofunction with Luetinizing Hormone and Thyroid Stimulating Hormone.

Practitioner Notes:

- The testes/ovaries, pituitary and hypothalmus are involved in an endocrine feed-back loop. This means there is often an advantage to designing nutrition for the whole system:
  M+ or F+ for gonads
  #1 for hypothalamus
  Gb for pituitary. - J.T.

Other Notes:

GAMMA GLOBULIN

Optimal (Clinical Nutrition) Values 0.8 - 1.5 g/100 ml.

Pathological (Lab) Reference Values: 0.5 - 1.5 g/100 ml.

Gamma Globulin: Is a class of antibodies concerned with chronic inflammation and auto immune activity.

Pathological Considerations:

Increased Gamma Globulin	
Carcinoid syndrome	OXCC, #5, Gt
Congestive heart failure	H, #5, Hcv
Dermatomyositis	#4, ACX, GOLD
Digestive inflammation	#3, AO, GOLD, DCSU
Hepatitis	L, Ls, #4, GOLD
Infections	GOLD, #3
Liver dysfunction	L, Ls, #5
Lupus, systemic eryth	OXCC, OXAA, #5, S
Micro-parasites	VRM-2, VRM-4, GOLD
Mononucleosis	L, Ls, VIVI, #4
Protein malnutrition	D, PRO

Decreased Gamma Globulin	
Adrenal cortex hyperfunction	Ga, Gb, PTM, Gt
Infection, chronic	#3, ATAK, OXOX, VIVI
Immunodeficiency	Gt, EV, S, ATAK
Renal dysfunction	K, Ks, #5
Respiratory distress	R, #3

Clinical Nutrition:

For Increased Gamma Globulin	
L	Liver
Ls	Liver Stimulant
#3	Anti-Infective
ATAK	Immune Rejuvenator

For Decreased Gamma Globulin	
L	Liver
Ls	Liver Stimulant
Gt	Thymus
Gf	Thyroid

Clinical Crossreference:

- **Adrenal Cortex Hyperfunction** = ↑ Gamma Glob. + ↓ Potassium (See Potassium)
- **Congestive Heart Failure** = ↑ Gamma Glob. + ↑ SGOT (See SGOT)
- **Dermatomyositis** = ↑ Gamma Glob. + ↑ Alpha 2 Glob. (See Alpha 2 Glob.)
- **Digestive Inflammation** = ↑ Gamma Glob. + ↓ Total Protein (See Total Protein)

- **Hepatitis** = ↑ Gamma Glob. + ↑ SGOT (See SGOT)
- **Immunodeficiency** = ↓ Gamma Glob. + ↓ Alb. + ↓ HCT + ↓ HGB + ↓ Total Protein + ↓ WBC + ↓ Platlets + ↓ Lymphs + ↑ MCV
- **Lupus, systemic erythmatosis** = ↑ Gamma Glob. + ↓ WBC (See WBC)
- **Micro-parasites** = ↑ Gamma Glob. + ↑ EOS (See EOS)

Related Tests:

Alpha 1 Globulin, Alpha 2 Globulin, Beta Globulin, Total Globulin, Total Protein

Clinical Notes:

- Parasites that can elevate Gamma Globulin include: histoplasmosis, schistosomiasis, stronglyoidasis, toxoplasmosis.

Practitioner Notes:

- Verify if adrenal cortex hypofunction is responsible for elevated Gamma Globulin values. - J.T.

Other Notes:

GAMMA-GLUTAMYL TRANSPEPTIDASE (GGTP)

Optimal (Clinical Nutrition) Values: 28 - 36 u/l.

Pathological (Lab) Reference Values: Men: 6 - 28 u/l
Women:

GGTP: Also listed by some labs as GGT, is an enzyme where activity is an early indicator of liver dysfunction. It is considered specific to the liver and usually elevates prior to Alkaline Phosphatase, SGOT, and SGPT but is also found in kidneys, prostate, and spleen. Evaluated bilirubin in the urine precedes GGTP as the earliest indicator of liver dysfunction. GGTP is particularly sensitive to alcohol intake and obstructive diseases and elevates quickly under such circumstances. Its enzyme function is to transport amino acids and peptides across cell membranes, and it is also involved in glutathione metabolism.

Pathological Considerations:

Increased GGTP	
Alcoholism	L, Ls, #6
Biliary obstruction	Lb, Ls
Cardiovascular abnormalities	Hcv, H, PTM MIN
Cholecystitis	Lb, #3, GOLD Ls
Cirrhosis	L, Ls, OXCC, OXAA, #5, 6
Diabetes Mellitus	L, Ls, P, Gb
Epilepsy	B, Hn, #5, L, Ls, #4
Hepatic, Biliary, Malignancy	L, Ls, OXCC, #5
Liver cell damage	L, Ls, #6, DSIR
Liver Disease	L, Ls, DSIR, #5
Mononucleosis	L, Ls, #4, CTV VIVI, ATAK
Myositis	KYRO, VRM-4, #3
Pancreatic Malignancy	P, OXCC, #5
Pancreatitis	P, #3, DSIR, D
Porphyria	L, Ls, OXAA, D
Post Radiation Therapy	L, Ls, Gf, ACX, Gt
Skeletal muscle damage	KYRO, #6, ACP
Trauma, severe	#6, AZV, MIN, Nc

Decreased GGTP	
Not clinically significant	
Vitamin A decreased	AZV
Vitamin K decreased	AZV

Clinical Nutrition:

For Increased GGTP	
L	Liver
Ls	Liver Stimulant
ACX	Vitamin Detox
D	Digestive

DSIR Digestant Internal Regenerator
Methionine

For Decreased GGTP	
LEV	Lecithin
BSV	Stress B-Vitamin
AZV	Multi-Vitamin

Methionine
Iodine (check for ↑ T4)

Clinical Crossreference:

- **Alcoholism** = ↑ GGTP + ↑ SGPT + ↑ SGOT + ↑ Alkaline Phosphase + ↑ Calcium + ↑ Copper + ↑ Bilirubin + ↑ CPK + ↑ FSH + ↑ LDH + ↑ PTH + ↑ Plasma ↑ Cortisol + ↑ Serum Phosphorus + ↑ Triglycerides + ↑ Uric Acid + ↓ Potassium + ↓ Plasma Phosphorus + ↓ Platelets
- **Biliary Obstruction** = ↑ GGTP + ↑ SGPT + ↑ SGOT + ↑ Acid Phos. + ↑ Triglycerides + ↑ Amylase + ↑ Bilirubin + ↑ Cholesterol + ↑ Globulin (Alpha 2, Beta) + ↑ WBC + ↑ LDH + ↑ Vitamin A + ↓ Vitamin K
- **Bone Disease** = Normal GGTP + ↑ Alk. Phos.
- **Developing Liver Pathology** = ↑ GGTP + ↑ SGPT + ↑ Alkaline Phosphatase
- **Fatty Liver Congestion** = ↓ GGTP + ↓ SGPT + ↓ Cholesterol
- **Hepatitis** = ↑ GGTP + ↑ SGOT + ↑ SGPT + ↑ WBC (+12,000)
- **Liver Disease** = ↑ GGTP + ↑ Alk. Phos. (See SGOT)

Related Tests:

Alkaline Phosphatase, Bilirubin, Cholesterol, CPK, LDH, SGOT, SGPT.

Clinical Notes:

- Pathological considerations for elevated GGTP are the same as elevated SGOT pathological considerations.
- Men generally have higher normals of GGTP due to its presence in the prostate.
- GGTP does not elevate in bone disorders, kidney failure, neonatal hepatitis, pregnancy, skeletal muscle disease.

Practitioner Notes:

- GGTP can help monitor the alcoholic's recovery program and serve as proof of compliance to a no-alcohol lifestyle. - J.T.

Other Notes:

GLOBULIN, TOTAL

Optimal (Clinical Nutrition) Values: 2.8 - 3.5 g/100 ml.

Pathological (Lab) Reference Values 2.0 - 4.2 g/100 ml.

Total Globulin: Is a combination of four globular proteins - Alpha 1, Alpha 2, Beta, and Gamma. Globulins function in antibody formation, coagulation, and play a role in maintaining the osmotic pressure of the blood since globulins are larger molecules than albumin and remain in the bloodstream. The specific fraction (s) of total globulin responsible for an altered lab report can be isolated by electrophoresis.

Pathological Considerations:

Increased Total Globulin	
Carcinoid syndrome	OXCC, #5, Gt
Digestive hypochlorhydria	D, #1, Ds
Hepatitis	L, Ls, #4, GOLD
Infections, bacterial	GOLD, #3, CTV
Infections, viral	VIVI, ATAK, #4
Liver dysfunctions	L, Ls, #5, #6
Malignancy, early	OXCC, #5, Gt
Parasites (Histoplasmosis, Schistomiasis)	VRM-3, VRM-4, WO
Rheumatoid arthritis	ARTA, SENG, #3
Typhoid fever	GOLD, ATAK

Decreased Total Globulin	
Anemias, severe	BSV, MIN, BLDB
Acute cholecystitis (gall bladder infection)	Lb, #3, DSIR
Acute hepatitis	L, Ls, #4, GOLD
Acute nephritis	K, #3, GOLD
Biliary cirrhosis	Lb, OXAA, OXCC, #5
Malnutrition	PRO, MIN
Multiple sclerosis	OXCC, Hn, LEV, CAL, EZV, FLX
Nephrosis	K, Ks, #5
Portal cirrhosis	Lb, OXAA, OXCC, #5

Clinical Nutrition:

For Increased Total Globulin	
D	Digestive
L	Liver
Ls	Liver Stimulant

For Decreased Total Globulin	
D	Digestive
L	Liver
Ls	Liver Stimulant
PRO	Nutro-Protein

Clinical Crossreference:

- **Anemias** = ↓ Globulin + ↓ RBC (See MCV)
- **Bacterial Infection** = ↑ Globulin + ↑ WBC (See WBC)
- **Digestive Hypochlorhydria** = ↑ Globulin + ↑ Alk. Phos. + ↓ CO_2 + ↓ Albumin + ↓ Calcium + ↓ Phosphorous + ↓ B-12 + ↓ Folates + ↑ Parathyroid Hormone
- **Hepatitis** = ↑ Globulin + ↑ SGPT + ↑ SGOT + ↑ GGTP (See GGPT)
- **Liver Dysfunction** = ↑ Globulin + ↑ SGPT + ↑ SGOT + ↑ GGTP (See SGPT)
- **Parasites** = ↑ Globulin + EOS (See EOS)
- **Rheumatoid Arthritis** = ↑ Globulin + ↑ Alk. Phos. (See Alk. Phos.)

- **Viral Infection** = ↑ Globulin + alt. WBC (See WBC)

Related Tests:

A/G Ratio, Alkaline Phosphatase, BUN/Creatinine Ratio, GGT, Glucose, LDH, Protein Electrophoresis, SGOT, Uric Acid.

Clinical Notes:

- Blood tests are not definitive for digestive hypochlorhydria.
- If an anemic trend is established, hypochlorhydria should be considered.

Practitioner Notes:

- An increased Total Globulin is generally indicative of inflammation (hepatitis, arthritis, colitis) or immune disorders. - J.T.
- A decreased Total Globulin is generally indicative of immune system insufficiency, liver disease, and excessive detoxification therapies. - J.T.

Other Notes:

GLUCOSE

Optimal (Clinical Nutrition) Values 85 - 100 mg/dl.

Pathological (Lab) Reference Values: 70 - 110 mg/dl.

Glucose: the bloodstream's sugar level, is the cell's main energy source. Too little glucose can result in hypoglycemia, too much can mean hyperglycemia (diabetes). Insulin from the pancreas controls the rate at which glucose is metabolized by the cells. Glucagon causes glycogen breakdown which elevates glycose levels. The liver controls the overall glucose levels of the blood. The thyroid sets the pace of liver function. The adrenals have a feedback loop to the pancreas to stop insulin secretion. The pituitary influences glucose levels by its effects on the liver. A fasting glucose over 110 should be viewed as a potential hyperglycemic (diabetic) trend. A fasting glucose level below 70 can be viewed with suspicion, but a 5-hour glucose tolerance test is needed to confirm hypoglycemia.

Pathological Considerations:

Increased Glucose	
Asthma	R, Ga, ACX, #6, 3, ATAK
Burns severe, first 24 hours	#6, AO, DSIR, DCSU
Cerebral lesions	B, #5
Coronary thrombosis	Hcv
Diabetes mellitus	P, Ls, L, Gb
Endocrine hyperfunction	G, Ga, Gf, Nc
Hyperpituitarism (early)	Gb, #5
Hyperthyroidism	Gf, #5, L, Ls
Infections	#3, GOLD, EV
Intercranial pressure, increased	Nc
Nephritis, chronic	K, #3, GOLD
Pituitary adenoma	Gb, #5, OXCC
Potassium deficiency	PTM
Pregnancy	L, Ps BSV
Shock	BLDB, Nc
Stress, Severe	Ga, Hn, MIN, BSV AZV
Uremia	K, Ks, ACX
Urinary obstruction	KDIR, K

Decreased Glucose	
Addison's disease	Ga, #5
Carcinoma of islet tissue	P, OXCC, #5
Endocrine Hypofunction	Gf, Gb, Ga, #1, #2
Glycogen storage disease	L, Ls
Hepatic insufficiency	L, Ls, #6
Hyperinsulinism (Hypoglycemia)	Ps, L, Ls, Ga #6, S
Hypoadrenalism	Ga, #1
Hypopituitarism (late)	Gb, #1
Hypothyroidism	Gf, #1, Gb
Insulin effect	*Chromium, Vanadium*
Liver destruction, excessive	L, Ls, Lb, #6, DSIR
Mumps	VIVI, #3, ACX
Pancreatic adenoma	P, OXCC, #5
Starvation (Starvation Diets)	PRO, AZV, MIN
Vomiting pregnancy, pernicious	BLDB, C, O, L

Clinical Nutrition:

For Increased Glucose	For Decreased Glucose
L Liver	**Ps Pancreas Stimulant**
Ls Liver Stimulant	**Ls Liver Stimulant**
P Pancreas	P Pancreas
ACX Vitamin Detox	L Liver
LEV Lecithin	Ga Adrenal
FLX Vegetable Omega-3 Flax Seed Oil	BLDB Blood Builder
CAL Calcium Plus	*Chromium*
PTM Potassium Stabilizer	
Chromium	
Zinc	
Vitamin B-6	

Clinical Crossreference:

- **Carbohydrate Utilization Poor** = ↑ Glucose
- **Diabetes Diathesis** = ↑ Glucose + ↑ Triglycerides + ↑ LDH + ↑ SGOT + ↑ Creat. + ↑ BUN + ↑ Chol + ↑ Uric Acid + ↑ Acid Phos.
- **Hypoglycemia, Possible** = ↓ Glucose + ↓ LDH
- **Liver Diabetic** = ↑ Glucose + ↑ SGPT + ↑ GGT + ↑ SGOT

Related Tests:

Alkaline Phosphate, CO_2, Cortisol, Creatinine, Electrolytes, Bilirubin, Glycohemoglobin, GTT, SGOT, Total Protein, Triglycerides.

Clinical Notes:

- Follow *Pro-Vita! Plan for Optimal Nutrition* dietarily.
- Glucose metabolism can become disordered if:
  1. ACTH is increased.
  2. Liver fails to breakdown glycogen.
  3. Glucose absorption is impaired in the intestines.
  4. Insulin receptors become reduced.
  5. Pancreas' beta cells decline reducing insulin production.

Warning: Glucose elevated above 140 mg/dl. is diagnostic of diabetes. Glucose elevated above 300 mg/dl. can cause a coma. Glucose under 30 mg/dl. can lead to brain damage.

Practitioner Notes:

- In hypoadrenalism, to augment Ga Adrenal supplementation, consider the special needs for the nutrients essential to adrenal hormone synthesis such as B-6, B-2, Pantothenic Acid, and Tyrosine. The building block of Tyrosine may suffice (Iron and Phenylalanine). Try the building blocks first before Tyrosine is tried. If a trial of Tyrosine is tried, the liver enzymes SGOT and SGPT should be checked prior to starting and again 30 days after. Typical doses range from 1500 - 2500 mg on arising on an empty stomach. If there is a history of birth control pills (3 or more months), a maintenance dose of B-6 (50 - 100 mg) should be considered to help the adrenals. - R.M.

- Increased Glucose is generally indicative of an underactive pancreas and overactive adrenals. - J.T.

- Decreased Glucose is generally indicative of overactive pancreas and underactive adrenals. J.T.

Other Notes:

HEMATOCRIT (HCT)

Optimal (Clinical Nutrition) Values: Male 41 - 49%, Female 37 - 46%

Pathological (Lab) Reference Values:
Adult Male 36 - 50%
Adult Female 34 - 44%
Children 31 - 41%
Newborns 44 - 64%

Hematocrit: Is a measurement of the volume of red blood cells in a portion of whole blood after it is centrifuged, and presents precise information for determining anemia (lack) or polycythemia (excess) of red blood cells. If fluids shift from the blood to the tissues, the RBC concentration increases, and if fluids hydrate into the bloodstream, the RBC concentration decreases.

Pathological Considerations:

Increased

Adrenal cortes, hyper	Ga, Gt
Anemia, B-6	BSV, BLDB
Dehydration	MIN
Diarrhea	WO, PTM
Emphysema	R, #5
Polycythemia	OXAA, #5
Respiratory Distress	R
Surgery	#6, BLDB

Decreased

Anemia, folic acid	BSV, BLDB
Anemia, iron	MIN, BLDB
Anemia, heredity	BSV, MIN, BLDB
Anemia, pernicious	BSV, BLDB
Carcinoid syndrome	OXCC, #5
Digestive inflam	D, #3, GOLD
Kidney dysfunction	K, Ks
Liver dysfunction	L, Ls, Lb
Malnutrition, protein	D, PRO
Parasites	VRM-1, 2, 3, 4
Rheumatoid arthritis	ARTA, SENG, #3
Ulcers, stomach & GI	DCSU, #6, AO

Clinical Nutrition:

For Increased

L	Liver
Ls	Liver Stimulant
S	Spleen

For Decreased

Gf	Thyroid
Gt	Thymus
S	Spleen
LEV	Lecithin
BLDB	Blood Builder

Clinical Crossreference:

- **Adrenal Cortex Hyperfunction** = ↑ HCT + ↓ K^+ (See Potassium)
- **Adrenal Cortex Hypofunction** = ↓ HCT + ↑ K^+ (See Potassium)
- **Anemia, Folic Acid** = ↓ HCT + ↑ MCV (See MCV)
- **Anemia, Pernicious** = ↓ HCT + ↑ MCV (See MCV)

- **Anemia, Vitamin B-6** = ↑ HCT + ↓ MCV (See MCV)
- **Diarrhea** = ↑ HCT + ↓ K^+ (See Potassium)
- **Digestive Inflammation** = ↓ HCT +↓ Total Protein (See Protein, total)
- **Kidney Dysfunction** = ↓ HCT + ↑ Creat. (See Creatinine)
- **Liver Dysfunction** = ↓ HCT + ↑ SGOT (See SGOT)
- **Parasties** = ↓ HCT + ↑ EOS (See EOS)
- **Protein Malnutrition** = ↓ HCT + ↓ Total Protein (See Protein, Total)
- **Rheumatoid Arthritis** = ↓ HCT + ↑ Alk. Phos (See Alk. Phos.)

Related Tests:

HGB, MCH, MCHC, MCV, RBC.

Clinical Notes:

- Increased HCT is often associated with spleen hyperfunction.
- Decreased HCT is often associated with thymus hyperfunction.
- HCT can help determine hydration when compared to Albumin and Globulin.

Practitioner Notes:

Other Notes:

HEMOBLOBIN (HGB)

Optimal (Clinical Nutrition) Values
Male 14.5 - 15.5 g/dl.
Female 13.5 - 15.0 g/dl.

Pathological (Lab) Reference Values:
Men 12 - 17 gm%, Women 11 - 15 gm%
Male: 14 - 18 g/dl.
Female: 12 - 16 g/dl.

Hemoglobin: Is the iron-containing protein found in red blood cells that carries oxygen from the lungs throughout the body and carbon dioxide (and other gasses) from the blood to the lungs for excretion. Heme is the pigmented, non-protein part of the hemoglobin made primarily in the liver but also in most other tissues. Heme is converted to hemoglobin in the bone marrow. In other tissues, heme is used for various metabolic processes.

The hemoglobin molecules ability to carry oxygen is determined by the pH (7.4 is optimal) the presence of ferrous iron, as well as the size and shape of the red blood cell.

Pathological Considerations:

Increased HGB/HCT	
Adrenal cortex, hyper	Ga, Gt
Anemia, B-6	BSV, BLDB
Asthma	R, Ga, ACX
Dehydration	MIN
Diarrhea	WO
Emphysema	R, #5
Polycythemia	OXAA, #5
Respiratory distress	R

Decreased HGB/HCT	
Adrenal cortex, hypo	Ga, #1
Anemia, folic acid	BSV, BLDB
Anemia, iron	BLDB, MIN, BSV
Anemia, pernicious	BSV, BLDB
Anemia, Vitamin C	CTV, MIN, BLDB
Carcinoid Tumors	OXCC, #5
Kidney dysfunction	K, Ks
Liver dysfunction	L, Ls
Malnutrition, protein	PRO, D
Parasites	VRM-1, 2, 3, 4
Rheumatoid arthritis	ARTA, SENG, #3
Ulcers, Stomach & GI	DCSU, #6, AO
Vitamin B-1 deficiency	BSV

Clinical Nutrition:

For Increased HGB/HCT

LEV	Lecithin
CTV	Vitamin C Therapy

S Spleen
Iron
Vitamin C
Copper

For Decreased HGB/HCT

Gf	Thyroid
Gt	Thymus
S	Spleen
LEV	Lecithin
BSV	Stress B Vitamin

Clinical Crossreference:

- **Adrenal Cortex Hyperfunction** = ↑ HGB + ↓ (K^+) See Potassium
- **Adrenal Cortex Hypofunction** = ↓ HGB + ↑ (K^+) See Potassium
- **Anemia, Iron Deficiency** = ↓ HGB + ↓ HCT + ↑ Bili. + ↓ Iron + ↓ MCV + ↓ MCHC + ↑ Glob. (above 2.8) + ↑ B-12
- **Asthma** = ↑ HGB + ↑ HCT + ↑ EOS + ↑ LDH + ↑ Neut. + ↑ SGOT + ↑ Uric Acid + ↓ (K^+) + ↓ Phos. + ↓ Lymph
- **Diarrhea** = ↑ HGB + ↓ (K^+)
- **Emphysema** = ↑ HGB + ↑ HCT + ↑ (K^+) + ↑ Ammonia + ↑ CO_2 + ↓ Phos. + ↓ Chlor. + ↓ Alpha Antitrypsin
- **Parasties** = ↓ HGB + ↑ EOS (See EOS)
- **Polycythemia** = ↑ HGB + ↑ HCT + ↑ Bili. + ↑ Platelets + ↑ EOS + ↑ WBC + ↑ Uric Acid + ↓ MCH + ↓ MCV + ↓ MCHC + ↓ Iron
- **Protein Malnutrition** = ↓ HGB + ↓ Total Protein (See Protein, total)
- **Respiratory Distress** = ↑ HGB + ↑ Total Protein (See Protein, total)

Related Tests:

HCT, MCH, MCHC, MCV, RBC.

Clinical Notes:

- A lack of exercise is often associated with elevated HGB/HCT/RBC.

Practitioner Notes:

- Aspirin use causes decreased HGB as well as iron imbalances. Thus, the advice to take an aspirin a day to prevent heart attacks is ill founded when viewed from the whole person perspective and what can be accomplished nutritionally. - J.T.

Other Notes:

IRON, TOTAL SERUM

Optimal (Clinical Nutrition) Values 85 - 110 mcg/dl.

Pathological (Lab) Reference Values: 40 - 200 mcg/dl.

Serum Iron: Is vital in red blood cell production as well as to spleen and liver activity. Iron is carried in the blood in the ferric form attached to a protein, siderophilin. Some iron is stored in the bone marrow and is used in the construction of red blood cells. Pregnant women and nursing mothers should pay special attention to their iron levels because they are susceptable to substantial iron loss. This test helps reveal iron deficiencies (anemia) or overloads (hemochromatosis).

Pathological Considerations:

Increased Serum Iron	
Aplastic anemia	BSV, BLDB, MIN
Hemolytic anemia	BSV, BLDB, MIN
Hepatitis	Ls, #4, L, GOLD
Hypochromatosis	BLDB
Intrinsic Factor low	PRO, D
Iron therapy, excessive	Reduce
Liver dysfunction	L, Ls
Pernicious anemia	BSV, BLDB, MIN
Primary marrow dysfunction	OXCC, #5, OXAA
Renal dysfunction	K, Ks, #5, #6

Decreased Serum Iron	
Chronic infections	Gt, #3, OXOX
Hypochromia anemia	BLDB
Liver Dysfunction	L, Ls
Nephrosis	K, #3
Pathological bleeding (GI tract)	OXCC, #5, DSIR
Renal Dysfunction	K, Ks, #5, #6
Uremia	K, #5
Vitamin C Deficiency	CTV

Clinical Nutrition:

For Increased Serum Iron

BLDB Blood Builder
BSV Stress B-Vitamin
MIN Multi-Mineral

Copper

For Decreased Serum Iron

BLDB Blood Builder
#1 Activator

CTV Vitamin C Therapy
S Spleen
M+ Male Endocrine; F + Female Plus
EZV Vitamin E 200

Clinical Crossreference:

- **Anemia, Folic Acid Deficiency** = ↑ Iron. + ↑ MCV + ↑ MCHC (See MCV)
- **Anemia, Iron Deficiency** = ↓ Iron + ↓ MCV + ↓ MCHC (See MCV)
- **Anemia, Pernicious (Vitamin B-12 Deficiency)** = ↑ Iron + ↓ MCV + ↓ MCHC (See MCV)
- **Anemia, Vitamin B-6 Deficiency** = ↑ Iron + ↓ MCV + ↓ MCHC (See MCV)
- **Deficiency In RBC Production** = ↑ Elevated Iron

- **Intrinsic Factor Deficiency** = ↑ Iron + ↓ H C T
- **Renal Dysfunction** = alt. Iron + ↑ Creatinine (See Creatinine)

Related Tests:

- Hemopoetic: Bilirubin, CBC, HCT, HGB, Ferritin, Transferrin.
- Liver Dysfunction: Alkaline Phos., GGT, LDH, SGPT.

Clinical Notes:

- Serum Iron values do not accurately reflect iron stores in the body.
- Iron values can decrease after menses.

Practitioner Notes:

Other Notes:

- Over 3/4 of the iron in the body is bound to hemoglobin, the substance in red blood cells that carries oxygen. All of the body's iron originates in food. Iron from old red blood cells is recycled. Men generally have sufficient stores of iron to last for years, even if it is not included in the diet. Women, on the other hand, need to replenish iron due to its loss in menstruation.

LACTIC DEHYDROGENASE (LDH)

Optimal (Clinical Nutrition) Values 120 - 160 iu/l

Pathological (Lab) Reference Values: 90 - 250 iu/l

Lactic Dehydrogenase: Is a group of enzymes found in blood and all tissues and is involved in carbohydrate metabolism. LDH participates in the conversion of pyruvic acid to lactate in the anerobic glycolysis of glucose. With the help of LDH, lactic acid can be converted to pyruvic acid and be accepted into the inner cell where it is converted to ATP for cellular fuel. The highest concentrations of LDH are found in the heart, liver, kidneys, brain, skeletal muscles and red blood cells. Damage to any of these areas will elevate LDH, but elevated LDH is not specific to one tissue. Further fractional tests, isoenzymes, are required to locate a specific tissue.

Pathological Considerations:

Increased Lactic Dehydrogenase

Artifact hemolyzed samples	(Invalid)
Cirrhosis	Ls, OXCC, #5
Congestive heart failure	H, Hcv, EZV, MIN
Dermatomyositis	GOLD, TR, XL
Diabetes	L, Ls, P, Gb
Hemolitic pernicious anemia	BSV, BLDB, MIN
Hemotological disorders	BLDB, Ls, L, Lb
Hepatitis, acute	L, Ls, #3
Hyperthyroidism	Gf, #1, Gb
Kidney dysfunction	K, Ks
Liver/Gall bladder dysfunction	L, Ls, Lb
Malignancy anywhere in body	OXCC, #5, OXAA
Mononucleosis, infectious	#4, VIVI, ACX
Muscular dystrophy	KYRO, #5
Myocardial infarction	H, Hn, Hcv, EZV
Myologenous leukemia	OXCC, #5, S
Pancreas dysfunction	P, Ps
Pancreatitis, acute	P, #3
Parasites, occasional	VRM 1, 2, 3, 4
Pneumonia	R, #3, VIVI
Pulmonary embolism	H, #6, HCV
Rheumatic corditis, acute	JACK, RESEARCH
Rheumatoid arthritis	ARTA, SENG, #3
Skelatal muscle disease	KYRO, #6
Tissue necrosis	ACX
Viral hepatitis	L, Ls, VIVI, #4

Decreased Lactic Dehydrogenase

Alkaline blood with water drawn from blood to muscle.

Carbohydrate metabolic dysf.	D, P
Pancreas dysfunction	P, #5
Radiation toxicity	ACX

Clinical Nutrition:

For Increased Lactic Dehydrogenase	
Ps	Pancreas Stabilizer
P	Pancreas
LEV	Lecithin
L	Liver
H	Heart
CAL	Calcium Plus
PTM	Potassium Stabilizer

Chromium
Zinc
Niacin
Vitamin B-3

For Decreased Lactic Dehydrogenase	
Ps	Pancreas Stabilizer
P	Pancreas
CTV	Vitamin C Therapy

Chromium
Zinc

Clinical Crossreference:

- **Acidic Blood With Water Drawn From Muscle To Blood** = ↑ LDH
- **Alkaline Blood With Water Drawn From Blood To Muscles** = ↓ LDH
- **Anemia, Consider** = ↑ LDH + ↓ HGB/HCT
- **Cardiac Dysfunction** = ↑ LDH + ↑ SGOT
- **Diabetic Diathesis** = ↑ LDH + ↑ Trig. + Normal Cholesterol
- **Hepatitis, Consider** = ↑ LDH + ↑ SGPT
- **Hypothyroidism** = ↑ LDH + ↓ T3 Uptake
- **Intestinal Parasites** = ↑ LDH + ↑ Eosinophils
- **Kidney Dysfunction** = ↑ LDH + ↑ Creat.
- **Liver/Gall Bladder Dysfunction** = ↑ LDH + ↑ SGPT/GGPT
- **Muscular Dystrophy, Consider** = ↑ LDH + ↑ CPK
- **Pancreatic Enzyme Deficiency** = ↑ LDH + ↓ Cal. + ↓ Trig.
- **Pulmonary Embolism** = ↑ LDH + ↑ Bilirubin + Normal SGOT
- **Rheumatoid Arthritis** = ↑ LDH + ↑ Alk. Phos.

Related Tests:

Albumin, Alkaline Phosphatase, CBC, Chloride, CPK, EKG, Glyco-Hemoglobin, PHI, SGOT, Total Protein.

Clinical Notes:

- LDH is elevated by over acid pH.

Practitioner Notes:

- LDH is primarily an indicator of carbohydrate metabolism. Increased LDH shows a carbohydrate intolerance; decreased LDH shows poor carbohydrate metabolism usually or a result of pancreatic enzyme deficiency. - J.T.

Other Notes:

LYMPHOCYTES (LYMPH)

Optimal (Clinical Nutrition) Values 25 - 40%

Pathological (Lab) Reference Values: 12 - 48%

Lymphocytes: Are leukocytes that are nongranulocytes and part of the white blood cell sysfem comprising 20 - 35% of the WBCs in circulation. They help destroy toxic products of protein metabolism and fight infections. There are 2 sub-types of lymphocytes. B-Lymphocytes (B-Cells) derived from the bone marrow and spleen and are involved in the antibody/antigen response, and T-Lymphocytes (T-Cells) originally derived from and dependent on thymus interaction. Due to the AIDS pandemic, further delineations of T-Cells has become commonplace such as T-helper, T-suppresser, T-8 etc. Lymphocytes originate from the spleen, lymph nodes, thymus, tonsils, and appendix.

Pathological Considerations:

Increased Lymphosites	
Adrenal cortex hypofunction ...	Ga, #1
Adrenal Cortical Insufficiency.....	Ga
Brucellosis	GOLD,
Congenital & Secondary Syphilis	GOLD, ATAK
Dengue Fever	VIVI, EV
Exophthalmic Goiter	Gf, OXCC, #5
Flu	VIVI, ATAK, ACX
Graves disease	Gf, OXCC, #5
Hepatitis, Infectious	L, Ls, GOLD, VIVI
Infection, bacterial	GOLD
Infection, viral	VIVI
Lympho Sarcosa	OXCC, OXAA, S
Lymphocytosis, Acute Infections	S, #3, GOLD
Metabolic Rejectivity Syndrome....	
Mononucleosis, Infectious	L, Ls, GOLD
Mumps	VIVI, ACX
Parasites	VRM-1, 2, 3, 4
Pertussis	R, #3, GOLD
Pituitary, anterior or hypo	Ga, #1
Ricket's	AZV, K, CAL
Rubella	VIVI, ACX
Scurvy	CTV
Thyrotoxicosis	Gf, OXCC, #5
Tuberculosis	R, ATAK

Decreased Lymphosites	
Adrenal cortex hyperfunction ..	Ga, Gt
Flu	VIVI, ATAK, ACX
Free radical pathologies	OXCC, #5, CTV
Hypogammaglobinemia	Gt, EV
Immune defficiency	ATAK, Gt #4
Immune Deficiency	Gt, ATAK
Infections, chronic	#3, OXOX, ATAK
Lupus, systemic eryth.	OXCC, #5, S
Viral Infections	VIVI

Clinical Nutrition:

For Increased Lymphocytes	For Decreased Lymphocytes
CTV Vitamin C Therapy	**Gt Thymus**
ACX Vitamin Detox	**ATAK Immune Rejuvinator**
GOLD Immune Plus	**#3 Anti-Infective**
#3 Anti-Infective	*Superoxide Dismutase*
Gt Thymus	*B12*
4 Day Rotation Diet	*Folic Acid*

Clinical Crossreference:

- **Flu** = Alt. Lymph + Alt. WBC (See WBC)
- **Infections, acute** = ↑ Lymph + ↑ WBC (See WBC)
- **Infections, chronic** = ↓ Lymph + ↓ WBC (See WBC)
- **Lupus** = ↑ Lymph + Alt. WBC (See WBC)
- **Parasites** = ↑ Lymph + ↑ EOS (See EOS)

Related Tests:

Baso, EOS, Mono, Neut., WBC

Clinical Notes:

- Lymphs can help determine if an infection is acute or chronic when compared to WBC and Neut.

Practitioner Notes:

- Elevated lymphs can be indicative of "leaky gut" syndrome where macromolecytes enter the blood stream and cause digestive leucocytosis. - J.T.

Other Notes:

MEAN CORPUSCULAR HEMOGLOBIN (MCH)

Optimal (Clinical Nutrition) Values MCH 27 - 31, micro-micro gms.

Pathological (Lab) Reference Values: 26 - 33 micro-micro gms.

:H: Is the weight of hemoglobin in one red blood cell. An increase or decrease in MCH helps differentiate een anemias either in itself or when compared with the Mean Corpuscular Volume (MCV).

Pathological Considerations:

Increased MCH

emia, pernicious	BLDB, BSV
emia, folid acid	BLDB, BSV
emias, hereditary	BLDB, BSV

Decreased MCH

Anemia, iron	BLDB, BSV, MIN
Anemia, vitamin B-6	BLDB, BSV
Free radical pathologies	OXCC, #5, CTV
Hypochlordria	D, MIN
Lead poisoning	CLNZ, CTV
Parasites	VRM-2, VRM-4
Rheumatoid arthritis	ARTA, SENG, #3
Vitamin C deficiency	CTV

Clinical Nutrition:

For Increased MCH

DB	Blood Builder
V	Stress B-Vitamin

For Decreased MCH

BLDB	Blood Builder
BSV	Stress B-Vitamin
MIN	Multi-Mineral
CTV	Vitamin C Therapy

S Spleen
Vitamin B-12
Folic Acid
Iron

nical Crossreference:

nemias = Alt. MCH (See MCV)

rthritis, Rheumatoid = ↓ MCH + ↑ Alk. Phos (See Alk. Phos)

ypochlorhydria = ↓ MCH + ↑ Glob. (See Glob.)

arasites = ↓ MCH, ↑ EOS (See EOS)

ated Tests:

, HGB, Iron, MCHC, MCV, RBC.

Clinical Notes:

- MCH is decreased in hypochromic anemia.
- MCH is increased in macrocytic anemia.
- Don't take natural Vitamin E and Iron at the same time.
- No tea, milk, eggs, or foods containing phytic acid (whole grains & cereals) with iron therapy.
- Folate deficiency is present in more than half of patients with megaloblastic anemia (disease of proximal ileum).
- Disease of distal ileum may result in B12 deficiency - also potassium chloride can alter intestinal pH and depress B12 assimilation.
- Potassium can depress B12 absorption.
- For Hemolytic & Oligocythemic Anemia use Vitamin E to help with excessive free radicals.

Practitioner Notes:

Other Notes:

MEAN CORPUSCULAR HEMOGLOBIN CONCENTRATE (MCHC)

Optimal (Clinical Nutrition) Values 32 - 35 U/100 ml. (%)

Pathological (Lab) Reference Values: 31.5 36 U/100 ml. (%)

MCHC: Is the percentage of the red blood cell occupied by hemoglobin. 100 ml. of packed red blood cells is measured for the concentration of hemoglobin.

Pathological Considerations:

Increased	
Anemia, folic acid	BSV, BLDB
Anemia, pernicious	BSV, BLDB
Anemia, hereditary	BSV, BLDB, MIN

Decreased	
Anemia, iron	BLDB, MIN
Anemia, vitamin B-6	BSV, BLDB
Free radical pathologies	OXCC, #5, CTV
Hypochlorhydria	D, MIN
Lead poisoning	CLNZ, CTV
Parasites	VRM-2, VRM-4
Rheumatoid arthritis	ARTA, SENG, #3, WO, Ga

Clinical Nutrition:

For Increased	
BLD	Blood Builder
BSV	Stress B-Vitamin

For Decreased	
BLDB	Blood Builder
BSV	Stress B-Vitamin
MIN	Multi-Mineral
S	Spleen

Clinical Crossreference:

- See MCV

Related Tests:

HCT, HGB, MCH, MCV, RBC

Clinical Notes:

- See MCH

Practitioner Notes:

Other Notes:

MEAN CORPUSCULAR VOLUME (MCV)

Optimal (Clinical Nutrition) Values 85 - 88 cu. microns

Pathological (Lab) Reference Values: 80 - 94 cu. microns

MCV: Measures the size (volume) of a single red blood cell. Deviations from normal size are indicative of anemias and help differentiate the kind of anemia when compared to MCH and MCHC.

Pathological Considerations:

Increased

Anemia, folic acid	BSV, BLDB
Anemia, pernicious	BSV, BLDB
Anemia, hereditary	BSV, BLDB, MIN

Decreased

Anemia, iron	BLDB, MIN
Anemia, vitamin B-6	BSV, BLDB
Free radical pathologies	OXCC, #5, CTV
Hypochlorhydria	D, MIN
Lead poisoning	CLNZ, CTV
Parasites	VRM-2, VRM-4
Rheumatoid arthritis	ARTA, SENG, #3, WO, Ga

Clinical Nutrition:

For Increased

BLDB	Blood Builder
BSV	Stress B-Vitamin

For Decreased

BLDB	Blood Builder
BSV	Stress B-Vitamin
MIN	Multi-Mineral

S Spleen
Vitamin B12
Folic Acid
Iron

Clinical Crossreference:

- **Anemia, Vitamin B-12** = ↑ MCV + ↑ MCH + ↑ EOS + ↑ LDH + ↑ Ind. Bili. + ↑ Gastrin + ↑ Copper + ↓ Alb. + ↓ RBC + ↓ Chol. + ↓ HCT + ↓ HGB + ↓ (K^+) + ↓ B-12 + ↓ Folate + ↓ Uric Acid
- **Anemia, Folic Acid** = ↑ MCV + ↑ MCH + ↑ Iron + ↑ LDH + ↑ Copper + ↑ Lymph + ↑ Bilirubin + ↓ Alk. Phos + ↓ (K^+) + ↓ Folate + ↓ Uric Acid + ↓ Platelets + ↓ RBC + ↓ HGB + ↓ HCT + ↓ Neut.
- **Anemia, Iron** = ↓ MCV + ↓ HGB (See HGB)
- **Anemia, Vitamin B-6** = ↓ MCV + ↓ MCH + ↓ HCT + ↓ WBC + ↓ Neut. + ↑ HGB + ↑ Mono. + ↑ Iron
- **Arthritis, Rheumatoid** = ↓ MCV + ↓ MCH + ↑ Alk. Phos. (See Alk. Phos.)
- **Hypochlorhydria** = ↓ MCV + ↓ MCH + ↑ Glob. (See Glob.)

- **Parasites** = ↓ MCV + ↓ MCH + ↑ EOS (See EOS)

Related Tests:

HCT, HGB, Iron, MCH, MCHC, RBC.

Clinical Notes:

- A lack of hydrochloric acid in the stomach will inevitably lead to low iron values and an anemic trend.

Practitioner Notes:

- A B-6 anemic trend may involve a zinc defficiency. Check for a decreased Alk. Phos. If Alk. Phos is decreased, zinc and B-6 should both be used. - J.T.

- Postmenstrual anemia is best supported with B-Complex, rather than just B-6 alone. - J.T.

Other Notes:

MONOCYTES

Optimal (Clinical Nutrition) Values 3 - 7%

Pathological (Lab) Reference Values: 2 - 8%

Monocytes: Are the largest of the white blood cells (WBC) and make up .5% to 10% of the total WBC count. They phagocytize micro organisms, particularly bacteria and protozoa, and various other non-self particles. In inflammatory processes, neutrophils (polys and segs) increase during the first three days, and the monos remain after that to clean up the cell fragments.

Pathological Considerations:

Increased Monocytes

Acute Infection, recovery	Gt, #3
Agranulocytosis, recovery	BLDB, S, DCSU
Anemia, Hemolytic	BLDB, MIN, BSV
Anemia, Hypochromic	BLDB, MIN, BSV
Arthritism, Rhematoid	ARTA, SENG, #3
Brucellosis	GOLD, #3
Carbon Tetrachloride poisoning	CLNZ, ACX, L, K
Chronic Amoebic Dysentery	VRM-3, WO
Free Radical Pathologies	OXCC, #5, CTV
Gaucher's Disease	Lb, D
Hodgkin's Disease	OXCC, S, #5
Kala-azar	Ls, S, GOLD, ATAK, VRM-2
Leukemia, Monocytic	OXCC, S, #5
Lupus Erthematosis	OXCC, OXAA, #5
Malaria	S, VRM-4, ATAK
Mononucleosis	L, Ls, GOLD
Mumps	VIVI, ACX
Myeloma, Multiple	OXCC, OXAA, #5
Oriental Sore	Ls, S, GOLD, ATAK, VRM-2
Parasites	VRM-1, 2, 3, 4
Prostate, benign hypertrophy	Mpc, #3
Rock Mountain Spotted Fever	GOLD, K
Subacute Bacterial Endocarditis	H, #3, GOLD
Trypanosomiasis	S, VRM-2, VRM-4, WO
Tuberculosis	R, #3, ATAK
Typhoid Fever	GOLD, S
Typhus	GOLD, #3, Gt

Decreased Monocytes

Decreases rarely seen

Clinical Nutrition:

For Increased Monocytes	
CTV	Vitamin C Therapy
GOLD	Immune Plus
Gt	Thymus

Vitamin A
Proteolytic Enzymes
Superoxide Dismutase

For Decreased Monocytes	
Gt	Thymus
S	Spleen

Clinical Crossreference:

- **Brucellosis** = ↑ Mono. + ↑ Alk. Phos. (See Alk. Phos.)
- **Infection, Acute** = ↑ Mono. + ↑ WBC (See WBC)
- **Hepatitis** = ↑ Mono. + ↑ SGPT + ↑ GGTP (See SGPT)
- **Mononucleosis** = ↑ Mono. + ↑ SGPT + ↑ GGTP (See SGPT)
- **Mumps** = ↑ Mono. + ↑ WBC (See WBC)
- **Parasites** = ↑ Mono. + ↑ EOS (See EOS)
- **Prostate, Benign Hypertrophy** = ↑ Mono. + ↑ Creat. (See Creat.)

Related Tests:

Baso, EOS, Lymph, Neut. WBC.

Clinical Notes:

- High doses of corticosteroids will depress monocytes.
- Always consider liver dysfunction when monocytes are elevated.
- Elevated monocytes, eosinophils, and basophils may be indicative of food allergies, "leaky-gut" and parasites. Confirm mononucleosis with other symptoms such as sore throat, fever, fatigue, and lymph gland enlargement.
- Elevated monocytes occur as a result of excessive tissue breakdown.

Practitioner Notes:

- Compare Mono. to ESR. This provides insights to potential liver dysfunction and degree of inflammation. - J.T.

Other Notes:

NEUTROPHILS

Optimal (Clinical Nutrition) Values 55 - 65%, (Band 0 - 1%)

Pathological (Lab) Reference Values:
Segmented: 50 - 70%

Neutrophils: The primary granulocyte also called "polymorphonuclear neutrophils (PMN)" and "segs" function as phagocytes, engulfing foreign matter and releasing enzymes to disable infectious organisms and metabolic wastes. Immature neutrophils are called "stabs" or "bands" due to their large nuclei. Their presence is an indication of the immune system's difficulty in overcoming a latent infection developing. The neutrophil count can help determine if an infection is acute or chronic.

Pathological Considerations:

Increased Neutrophils (Neutrophilia)

Adrenal dysfunction	Ga
Allergies	Ga, ACX, CTV
Burns	#6, AO
Convulsions	MIN, #6
Coronary Thrombosis	HCV, OXCC
Diabetic Acidosis	L, Ls, P, Gb
Diptheria	#3, ACX
Eclampsia	PRO, Nc, K
Flu	VIVI, ACX, CDST
Gout	K, #5, PTM
Heart attack	H, #6, HCV
Hemolysis of Erthrocytes	BLDB, S, Gt
Infections, Acute bacterial	GOLD, ATAK, EV
Infections, Localized, pus	OXOX, #3, WO, ACX, GOLD
Malignant Neoplasms	OXCC, #5
Moribund Condition	
Paroxysmal Tachycardia	Hn, Hcv, EE
Poisoning, chemical, drug	ACX, CTV, CLNZ
Polycythemia	OXAA, #5
Postoperative	#6, AZV, MIN
Rheumatic Fever	Hn, S, GOLD, #3
Rheumatoid Arthritis	ARTA, SENG, #3
Severe Pain	N-3, KYRO
Smallpox	VIVI, ATAK, Gt
Stress	Hn, Ga, MIN
Uremia	Ks, K, #5

Decreased Neutrophils (Neutropenia)

Anemia, iron	BLDB, MIN
Bone Marrow Depression	OXAA
Folic acid deficiency	BSV, AZV
Infections, chronic	GOLD, #3, OXCC ATAK
Lupus erythmatosus	OXCC, #5, S, ATAK
Radiation therapy	Gt, ACX, CTV
Viral infection	VIVI
Vitamin B-6 deficiency	BSV, AZV
Vitamin B-12 deficiency	BSV, AZV

Clinical Nutrition:

For Increased Neutrophils	
# 3	Anti-Infective
GOLD	Immune Plus
Gt	Thymus
S	Spleen
CTV	Vitamin C Therapy
CAL	Calcium Plus
LEV	Lecithin
Vitamin A	

For Decreased Neutrophils	
# 3	Anti-Infective
Gt	Thymus
S	Spleen
CTV	Vitamin C Therapy
CAL	Calcium Plus
ATAK	Immune Rejuvenator

Clinical Crossreference:

- **Adrenal Dysfunction** = ↑ Neut + Alt. Potassium
- **Gout** = ↑ Neut. + ↑ Uric Acid (See Uric Acid)
- **Infection, Acute** = ↑ Neut. + ↑ WBC (See WBC)
- **Infection, Chronic** = ↓ Neut + ↓ WBC (See WBC)
- **Lupus** = ↓ Neut. + ↓ WBC (See WBC)
- **Rheumatoid Arthritis** = ↑ Neut. + ↑ Alk. Phos. (See Alk. Phos.)

Related Tests:

Baso, EOS, Lymphs, Mono, WBC.

Clinical Notes:

- An increase in mature neutrophils is often called a "shift to the right." An increase in immature (stab or band) neutrophils is often called a "shift to the left."
- Bone marrow depression can also indicate infection.
- Band cells indicate a latent infection developing in the system.
- Toxic drugs or prolonged infections, netrophils may become exhausted and the blood test will be low.
- Strenous physical exercise can temporarily elevate neutrophils, as does pregnancy and labor.
- Calcium is required to build a strong phagocyte, thus calcium assists neutrophil function.

Warning:

- A low (less than 500) neutrophil count predesposes a person to bacterial infections. Take preventative measures.

Practitioner Notes:

- In massive or prolonged infections, neutrophils may become exhausted and the blood test will be low. - J.T.

Other Notes:

PARATHYROID HORMONE (PTH)

Optimal (CN) Values, Furds Lab: 0.5 - 2.0 ng/ml

Pathological (Lab) Reference Values:
N-term 230 - 630 pg/ml
C-term 410 - 1760 pg/ml

Parathyroid Hormone: Is a polypeptide chain of 84 amino acids secreted by the parathyroid gland. Like the hormone insulin that is responsive to blood levels of a specific substance, and unlike most endocrine gland secretions which are responsive to other hormones, PTH is released based on the concentration of free calcium ions. Low levels of free calcium ions cause PTH to be secreted; high levels inhibit PTH secretion.

PTH acts on two tissues, bone and kidney, to influence the plasma free ionized calcium levels. Its action on bone is to stimulate the osteoclast cells to release calcium and phosphate into the lymph resulting in higher concentrations of plasma calcium and phosphate, and lower levels of calcium in the bones. Its action on the kidneys is to reduce phosphate by causing the renal tubules to decrease reabsorption of phosphate and have it pass out in the urine, resulting in an elevation of calcium ions uninhibited by phosphate.

Calcitonin is a thyroid hormone that modifies the action of PTH, thus it is antagonistic to PTH. Calcitonin causes calcium to enter the bone and thus lowers plasma levels. Together, Calcitonin and PTH maintain calcium homeostasis.

Pathological Considerations:

Increased PTH	
Hyperparathyroidism	Gf, Gb, CAL, K

Decreased PTH	
Hypoparathyroidism	Gf, Gb, BSV, K

Clinical Nutrition:

For Increased PTH	
Gf	Thyroid
Gb	Pituitary
CAL	Calcium Plus
K	Kidney

For Decreased PTH	
Gf	Thyroid
Gb	Pituitary
BSV	Stress B-Vitamin
K	Kidney

Clinical Crossreference:

- **Hyperparathyroidism** = ↑ PTH + ↑ Cal. + ↑ Uric Acid + ↑ Creat. + ↑ Gastrin + ↑ CO_2 + ↑ Alk. Phos. + ↑ Chlor. + ↑ Acid Phos. + ↓ Phos. + ↓ Trig. + ↓ Chol. + ↓ Mag.

- **Hypoparathyroid** = ↓ PTH + ↓ Alk. Phos. + ↓ Cal. + ↑ Phos. + ↑ Uric Acid

Related Tests:

Calcium, Phosphorus

Clinical Notes:

- Calcium can be depleted due to an over acid pH because it will be used to buffer the acids in the bloodstream.

- Excessive PTH levels can cause bone pain and nodosities.

Practitioner Notes:

- The following factors all play an important role in maintaining a positive calcium balance:

  * Normal parathyroid function (PTH)
  * Normal thyroid function (Calcitonin)
  * Normal kidney function (tubule filtration, Vitamin D-3)
  * Good digestion (HCI)
  * Adequate dietary intake of vegetable source calcium
  * Adequate dietary intake of Vitamin D
  * Proper pH cycles and maintenance of alkaline reserve
  * Exclusion of intake of substances that inhibit or deplete calcium including: sodas, coffee, steroid drugs, antibiotics, excessive red meat.
  * Adequate exercise (stimulates bone density)

  See *Osteoporosis: The Preventable Disease* listed in the catalog for more information. - J.T.

Other Notes:

PHOSPHORUS (PO4)

Optimal (Clinical Nutrition) Values 3.2 - 3.9 mg%

Pathological (Lab) Reference Values: 2.0 - 4.5 mg%

Phosphorus: Is an element required for bone growth and energy metabolism. Several factors are involved in the regulation of serum, inorganic, phosphorus including Parathyroid Hormone (PTH), Vitamin D, and the kidneys. Like potassium, phosphorus enters the cells assisted by the presence of insulin. There is a reciprocal relationship between phosphorus and calcium. The increase of one can cause a decrease of the other. PTH secretion is governed by the level of free ionic calcium in the blood, and one of its roles is to increase blood calcium and lower blood phosphorus levels. Low levels of free ionic calcium increase PTH and the excretion of phosphorus elevates. Responsive to PTH, the kidneys excrete phosphorus in the form of phosphates when PTH reduces the re-absorption of phosphate from the glomular filtrate. Most of the body's Phosphorus is stored in the bones as calcium phosphate. In addition to its role in bone physiology, Phosphorus is important for the formation of Phospholipids, ATP, Creatine, Phosphate, nucleic acids, and glucose utilization.

Pathological Considerations:

Increased Phosphorus	
Acromegaly	Gb, #5
Fracture Healing	MIN, CAL, #6, AZV, AO
Hypervitaminosis (D)	(Reduce)
Hypoparathyroidism	Gf
Nephritis	K, Gold, #3
Pituitrin Administration, After	
Renal insufficiency	K, KS
Renal Rickets	K, KDIR
Starvation	PRO, AZV, MIN
Uremia	Ks, K, #5

Decreased Phosphorus	
Alcoholism, Acute	AZV, MIN, L
Diabetes	P, L, Ls, Gb
Digestive Dysfunction	P, D
Hyperinsulin (Hypoglycemia)	Ps
Hyperparathyroidism	Gf, CAL
Hypopituitary	Gb, #1
Idiopathic Steatorrhea	D, Lb
Liver dysfunction	L, Ls, #5
Lobar Pneumonia	R, #3, Gold
Myxedema	Gf, #1, Gb
Neurofibromatosis	OXCC, #5, Hn
Osteomalacia	CAL, MIN, AZV
Ovary hypofunction	F+, Mpr, #1
Rickets	AZV, CAL, MIN, LEV
Sprue	DCSU, DSIR, AO
Vitamin D Deficiency	AZV

Clinical Nutrition:

For Increased Phosphorus

BSV Stress V-Vitamin

Hydrochloric Acid
Folic Acid
B12
Acidophilus Yeast
Bile Salts

For Decreased Phosphorus

MIN Multi-Mineral
AZV Multi-Vitamin

P Pancreas
Vitamin D
Comfrey-Pepsin
Acidophilus Yeast

Clinical Crossreference:

- **Digestive Hypochlorhydria** = ↓ Phos. + ↑ Total Protein + ↑ Total Globulin (See Globulin, Total)
- **Duodenal pH Decreased With Lack Of Pancreatic Bicarbonate** = ↓ Phos.
- **Fat Absorption, Poor** = ↓ Phos. + ↓ Calcium + ↓ Bilirubin
- **Gall Bladder Emulsification, Poor** = ↑ Phos. + ↓ Calcium
- **Gastric Intrinsic Problem, Possible** = ↓ Phos. + ↑ Calcium
- **Hyper-Vitaminosis Or Hydrochloric Acid Deficiency** = ↑ Phos. + ↑ Calcium
- **Hyperparathyroidism** = ↓ Phos + ↑ PTH
- **Hypoparathyroidism** = ↑ Phos. + ↓ PTH
- **Renal Dysfunction** = ↑ Phos. + ↑ Creat.
- **Vitamin D Deficiency** = ↓ Phos. + ↓ Calcium + ↑ Alk. Phos.

Related Tests:

Alkaline Phosphatase, Calcitonin, Gastric HCL, Serum Calcium, Total Protein.

Clinical Notes:

- The optimum Calcium/Phosphorus Ratio = 2.5/1.
- An indicator of intestinal pH. Low Phosphorus = Acid. High Phosphorus = Alkaline
- It is not uncommon for clinicians to apply the same supplemental therapy for both increased and decreased phosphorus.
- Excessive Vitamin D intake will elevate serum phosphorus and cause poor fatty acid utilization which in turn reduces ionic calcium.
- Supplemental adjustment of phosphorus must not occur at the expense of calcium.

Practitioner Notes:

- Soft drinks (sodas) contain phosphoric acid that elevates phosphorus at the expense of calcium. People who use sodas regularly jeopardize the calcium-phosphorus balance. - J.T.
- High protein diets cause elevation of phosphorous. - J.T

Other Notes:

PLATELETS

Optimal (Clinical Nutrition) Values 200,000 - 300,000/cu.mm

Pathological (Lab) Reference Values: 250,000 - 500,000/cu.mm

Platelets: Also called "Thrombocytes" are cells produced in the bone marrow by large polypoid cells called "megakarocytes". Platelets are concerned with blood clotting and dissolution of blood clots. Like red blood cells, platelets do not have nuclei, but platelets are only one fourth as large. The role of platelets in health is to protect the body and blood vessels from ruptures and bleeding. High in phospholipids, platelets are activated by calcitonin and combine with the proteins in collagen, elastin to seal off escaping blood and protect the damage area while repair is made.

Pathological Considerations:

Increased Platelets	
Anemias	BLDB, MIN, BSV
Blood clotting function low	LEV
Free radical pathologies	OXCC, #5, CTV
Polycythemia Vera	OXAA, #5
Rheumatoid arthritis	ARTA, SENG, #3

Decreased Platelets	
Anemias	BLDB, MIN, BSV
Free radical patholgies	OXCC, #5, CTV
Leukemia	OXCC, OXAA, S
Liver cirrhoris	L, Ls, OXCC
Lupus, systemic eryth.	OXCC, #5, S
Rubella	VIVI, ACX
Thrombocytopevic purpura	BLDB, S

Clinical Nutrition:

For Increased Platelets

- LEV Lecithin

For Decreased Platelets

- LEV Lecithin
- FLX Flax Seed Oil
- BLDB Blood Builder

Vitamin T

Clinical Crossreference:

- **Arthritis, rhematoid** = ↑ Plat. + ↑ Alk. Phos (See Alk. Phos.)
- **Cirrhosis, Liver** = ↓ Plat. +↑ SGOT, ↑ GGTP (See SGOT)
- **Lupus** = ↓ Plat. + ↓ WBC (See WBC)

Related Tests:

HCT, HGB, MCH, MCHC, MCV, RBC.

Clinical Notes:

- Vitamin T is found in sesame seeds.

Practitioner Notes:

- When free radicals damage an artery, platelets help put a patch over the leision to protect against rupture. If the blood contain excessive LDL cholesterol an excessively large patch may clump together and clog the artery or contribute to arteriosclerosis. - J.T.

Other Notes:

POTASSIUM (K^+)

Optimal (Clinical Nutrition) Values: 4.0 - 4.6 mEq./l.

Pathological (Lab) Reference Values: 3.5 - 5.0 mEq./l.

Potassium: (K^+)Is an electrolyte (positively charged mineral) that helps regulate the heart and other muscles in the body. It is chiefly an intracellular ion so serum potassium values only reflect a small (2%), but vital, amount of the body's total potassium. Potassium regulates the enzymes responsible for carbohydrate metabolism. Potassium plays a critical role in nerve conduction, muscle contraction, acid/alkaline balance, osmotic pressure, adrenal function and intracellular pH. Deficiencies in potassium are quite common but should not be evaluated by low serum potassium alone.

Pathological Considerations:

Increased Potassium	
Acidosis, metabolic	Ga, CAL
Addison's disease	Ga, #5
Adrenal Cortex Hypofunction	Ga, #1
Asthma, acute bronchial	R, Ga, ACX, #3 ATAK
Bradycardia	Hn, H
Diabetes	P, Ls, L, Gb
Diarrhea	WO, GOLD
Infections, acute	GOLD, #3
Pneumonia	R, #3, #4, GOLD, VIVI, ATAK
Renal dysfunction	K, Ks, ACX
Respiratory dysfunction	R
Tissue destruction	#6, ACP, PRO, MIN
Uremia	K, Ks, ACX

Decreased Potassium	
Anemia	BLDB, MIN, BSV, #S
Cramps	CAL, PTM, EE
Diarrhea, severe acute	WO, GOLD
Diuretics	PTM, *Mag.*, Ga
Hypercorticoadrenalism	Ga, Gb, PTM, Gt
Hyperinsulinism and diabetes	P, Ls, Gb
Hypertension	HCV, Nc, PTM
Intestinal alkalosis, congenital	APHA, BIF, C, PTM Ga
Junk Food Diet	Pro-Vita! Plan, PTM
Malignant growth	OXCC, #5, OXAA
Nephritis, chronic	K, #3, GOLD
O.D. of desoxycorticosterone	Ga, #6
O.D. of testosterone	Ga, M+
Paralysis, periodic, hereditary	N-3, #5
Primary aldosteronism	Ga, PTM
Sprue and chronic diarrhea	DCSU, D, PTM, DSIR, GOLD, AO

Clinical Nutrition:

For Increased Potassium

EZV Vitamin E
Ga Adrenal
Gb Pituitary
H Heart

DIJS Stomach Antacid

For Decreased Potassium

H Heart
Gb Pituitary
PTM Potassium Stabilizer

BSV Stress B-Vitamin
Hcv Cardio Vascular
MIN Multi-Mineral
Banana, Tomato

Clinical Crossreference:

- **Adrenal Cortex Hyperfunction** = ↓ (K^+) + ↑ (Na^+) + ↑ Chlor. + ↑ Cortisol + ↑ Aldosterone + ↑ (CO_2) + ↓ Renin
- **Adrenal Cortex Hypofunction** = ↑ (K^+) + ↑ Renin + ↓ (Na^+) + ↓ Chlor. + ↓ (CO_2) + ↓ Cortisol + ↓ Aldosterone
- **Congested Heart Cells** = ↑ (K^+)
- **Respiratory Dysfunction** = ↑ (K^+) + ↑ Total Protein (See Protein, Total)

Related Tests:

ACTH, Alkaline Phosphatase, BUN, Cortisol, Creatinine, EKG, Sodium.

Clinical Notes:

- Since serum potassium is only 2% of the body's total potassium, it can be an error to supplement potassium solely on a serum deficiency.
- Serum potassium elevates .6 mEq/l for every .1 drop in serum pH.
- The more effective form of potassium is organic (co-valent) potassium (potasium bitartrate) derived from grapes.
- Potassium levels prompt the pituitary (posterior) to regulate renal osmolality and specific gravity. It is the body's primary oxidizing mineral controlled by the posterior pituitary.

Warning:

- Potassium less than 2.5 m/Eq can result in heart failure. Potassium greater than 6.5 m/Eq can result in heart failure.

Practitioner Notes:

- A potassium deficiency will cause low protein synthesis. - J.T.
- An increased K^+ implies adrenal fatigue; a decreased K^+ implies over stimulated adrenals. - J.T.

Other Notes:

PROTEIN, TOTAL

Optimal (Clinical Nutrition) Values: 7.1 - 7.6 ml.

Pathological (Lab) Reference Values 6.6 - 8.3 ml.

Total Protein: The proteins in blood plasma are albumin. globulin. and fibrinogen. Collectively, these are total protein. Albumin and globulin are chiefly responsible for the colloidal osmotic pressure between plasma and tissue fluids. Albumin is the largest contributor to total protein. Hyperproteinemia is usually caused by a rise in one of the immunoglobins (Alpha 1, Alpha 2, Beta, Gamma). Hypoproteinemia results in edema and usually the albumin drops more profoundy than does Globulin. If albumin is low and total protein high, an immunoglobin assay and/or electrophoresis would better determine the implications.

Pathological Considerations:

Increased Total Protein	
Adrenal Cortex Hypofunction	Ga, #1
Anhydremia (dehydration)	MIN, AZV
Carcinoma (early)	OXCC, #5, GT
Diabetic Acidosis	P, CAL, Ga
Hypochlorhydria	D, Ds
Liver Dysfunction	L, Ls, #6, #5
Multiple Myeloma	OXCC, #5, OXAA
Pneumonia	R, #3, VIVI, GOLD, #4
Respiratory Disease	R, OXCC, HCV, #5
Rheumatoid Arthritis	ARTA, SENG, #3, WO

Decreased Total Protein	
Adrenal Cortex Hyperfunction	Ga, #6
Anemia	BLDB, MIN, BSV
Anovulatory Drugs	F+, L, Ls
Cardiac Edema	H, KDIR
Cirrhosis	L, Ls, OXCC, OXAA, #6, #5
Cretinism	B, Gb, I
Digestive Inflamation	D, GOLD, DCSU
Glomerulonephritis	K, #3, Ks
Hypertension, Essential Benign	HCV, PTM, MIN
Hyperthyroidism	Gf, Gb, #5
Infectious Hepatitis	L, Ls, #4, GOLD
Leukemia	OXCC, OXAA, #5, Gt, ATAK
Liver dysfunciton	L, Ls, #5, #6
Malnutrition	PRO, MIN
Myxedema	PRO
Nephrosis (renal dysfunction)	K, Ks, #5, #6
Pregnancy	PRO, MIN
Simmonds's Disease	Gb, F+, OXCC, Ga, Gf

Clinical Nutrition:

For Increased Total Protein

Gt	Thymus
D	Digestive
CAL	Calcium Plus
Gb	Thyroid

Ps Pancreas Stabilizer
SENG Red Ginseng
Iodine (Check T3, T4, T7)
Vitamin D

For Decreased Total Protein

LEV	Lecithin
L	Liver
Ls	Liver Stimulant
ACX	Vitamin Detox

PRO Nutro-Protein
BSV Stress B-Vitamin
Ds Digest Stabilizer
MIN Multi-Mineral
Niacin

Clinical Crossreference:

- **Adrenal Hyperfunction** = ↓ Protein + ↑ Potassium
- **Adrenal Hypofunciton** = ↑ Protein + ↓ Potassium
- **Digestive Inflamation** = ↓ Total Protein + ↓ Albumin + ↓ HCT/HGB + ↓ Lympho + ↓ B-12 + ↓ Cal + ↓ Globulin + ↓ Sodium + ↓ Potassium + ↓ MCH/MCHC + ↑ MCV + ↑ Uric Acid + ↑ BASO + ↑ EOS + ↑ Gamma Iso-fraction + ↑ Polys
- **Gastritis/Colitis** = ↓ Total Protein + ↓ Albumin + ↓ HCT/HGB + ↓ Lympho + ↓ B-12 + ↓ Cal + ↓ Globulin + ↓ Sodium + ↓ Potassium + ↓ MCH/MCHC + ↑ MCV + ↑ Uric Acid + ↑ BASO + ↑ EOS + ↑ Gamma Iso-Fraction + ↑ Polys = **Digestive Inflamation (Gastritis, Colitis, etc.)**
- **High Protein Diet** = ↑ Protein + ↑ A/G Ratio + ↑ Cholesterol
- **Hypertension, Benign Essential** = ↓ Total Protein + ↑ CO_2 + ↑ Uric Acid + ↑ BUN + ↑ Triglycerides + ↑ Renin + ↓ Potasium + ↓ Albumin + ↓ Sodium
- **Pancreatic Enzyme Deficiency** = ↑ Protein + ↑ Uric Acid + Altered Calcium
- **Poor Protein Assimilation** = ↓ Protein + ↓ Calcium
- **Protein Malnutrition** = ↓ Total Protein + ↓ BUN + ↓ HCT/HGB + ↓ Alb. ↓ WBC + ↓ Iron + ↓ CAL + ↓ Mag + ↓ Potassium + ↓ Alk. Phos. + ↓ Beta/Gamma Globulin + ↑ B-12 + ↓ A/G Ratio
- **Protein Metabolism, Depressed Due To Hepatic Insufficiency** = ↓ Protein + ↓ BUN + Altered SGPT
- **Renal Dysfunction** = ↓ Protein + ↑ Creatinine (See Creatinine)
- **Respiratory Inflamation And Distress** = ↑ Total Protein + ↑ BUN + ↑ Uric Acid + ↑ Potassium + ↑ Triglycerides + ↓ Bilirubin + ↓ Cortisol + Alt. Chlorides
- **Rheumatoid Arthritis** = ↑ Protein + ↑ Alk. Phos. (See Alk. Phos.)

Related Tests:

A/G Ratio, Alkaline Phosphatase, BUN, BUN/Creatinine Ratio, Calcium, GGTP, Glucose, Magnesium, SGOT, SGPT, Uric Acid.

Clinical Notes:

- Edema occurs when the serum protein level falls below 5 gm.%.
- *Follow Pro-Vita! Plan for Optimal Nutrition* dietarily (See Catalog).

Practitioner Notes:

Other Notes:

RED BLOOD CELL COUNT (RBC)

Optimal (Clinical Nutrition) Values 4.7 - 5.4 million/cu.mm

Pathological (Lab) Reference Values:
Men 4.1 - 5.6 million/cu.mm
Women 3.8 - 5.1 million/cu.mm

RBC: Mature erythrocytes (red blood cells) make up around 40% of the blood's volume averaging 30 trillion cells in an adult. The RBC imports oxygen from the lungs on its hemoglobin molecule and exports carbon dioxide and other waste-gasses back out through the lungs. If the RBC count is too low, there is not enough oxygen. If there are too many RBCs as in polycythemia, there is an inceased risk of blockage of capilaries. Basically, the RBC count helps determine the oxygen-carrying capacity of the blood.

Pathological Considerations:

Increased	
Adrenal cortex hyperfunction	Ga, Gt, Gb
Cystic fibrosis	R, #3, D, APHA
Dehydration	MIN
Emphasema	R, #5
Heart diseases, chronic	H, Hcv
Poisoning, acute	WO, ACX
Polcythemia, Vero	OXAA, #5
Pulmonary fibrosis	H, OXCC
Respiratory distress	R, Hcv, ACX

Decreased	
Anemias, many	BLDB, MIN, BSV
Carcinoid tumors	OXCC, #5
Hemorrhage, post	BLDB
Kidney dysfunction	K, Ks
Leukemia	OXCC, S, #5
Liver dysfunction	L, Ls

Clinical Nutrition:

For Increased

S Spleen
LEV Lecithin

Vitamin A
Vitamin E
Copper

For Decreased

LEV Lecithin
S Spleen PRO Nutro-Protein
BLDB Blood Builder

ACP Vitamin ACP

Clinical Crossreference:

- **Adrenal Cortes Hyperfunction** = ↑ RBC + ↑ Potassium (See Potassium)
- **Emphasema** = ↑ RBC + ↑ HGB (See Hemoglobin)
- **Anemias, Folic Acid** = ↓ RBC + ↑ MCV (See Mean Corpuscular Volume)
- **Anemia, Iron** = ↓ RBC + ↓ HGB (See Hemoglobin)
- **Anemia, Vitamin B-6** = ↓ RBC + ↓ MCV (See Mean Corpuscular Volume)
- **Liver Dysfunction** = ↓ RBC + ↑ SGPT + ↑ GGTP (See SGPT)

- **Kidney Dysfunction** = ↓ RBC + ↑ Creat. (See Creat.)
- **Respiratory Distress** = ↑ RBC + ↑ Total Protein (See Total Protein)

Related Tests:

MCH, MCHC, MCV, HGB, HGT.

Clinical Notes:

- RBCs are responsible for the red color of blood.
- A pH of 7.46 is optimal for hemoglobin transport of oxygen.

Practitioner Notes:

Other Notes:

SERUM GLUTAMIC-OXALACETIC TRANSAMINASE (SGOT) also (AST)

Optimal (Clinical Nutrition) Values 18 - 22

Pathological (Lab) Reference Values: 0 - 40

SGOT: A cytoplasmic enzyme found in the liver, heart, kidneys, brain, and skeletal muscles. SGOT is also called "AST" for Aspartate Aminotransferase because it acts as a catylist in amino acid metaolism during glycolysis resulting in energy release of the many transaminase enzymes, only SGOT and alanine aminotransferase (ALT) show increased activity in the blood as a result of liver, heart and skeletal muscle disease. SGOT is involved in the transfer of d-amino mintrogen of aspartic acid to alphaketoglutamic acid resulting in the synthesis of glutamic acid, oxaloecetic acid and alph-kefo acid.Injury related elevations of SGOT occur within ten hours of an injury, reaches a peak within thirty hours, and returns to normal levels within six days.

Pathological Considerations:

Increased SGOT	
Alcoholism	L, Ls
Arthritis, rheumatoid	ARTA, SENG, #3
Asthma	R, ACX, Ga
Brucellosis	GOLD, #3
Cirrhosis	L, Ls, #6, OXCC
Congestive heart failure	H
Diabetes	L, Ls, P, Gb
Free-Radical pathologies	L, Ls, CTV, EZV
Hemolytic jaundice	S, BLDB, L
Hepatitis, acute	L, Ls, #4, #3
Hepatocellular damage	L, Ls, #6
Hypertension, essential	Hcv
Infections, some	GOLD, #3, VIVI
Influenza	VIVI, ATAK
Intrahepatic neoplasma	OXAA, Ls, Ls, OXCC
Mononucleosis	L, Ls, #4, #3
Mononucleosis, infectious	L, Ls, VIVI, GOLD
Muscular dystrophy	OXCC, KYRO, #5
Mycardial infarction	H, #6
Myocarditis	VIVI, H, #3, GOLD
Myositis	KYRO, #6, VRM-4
Pancreatitis	P, #3
Parasites, occasional	VRM-1, VRM-3
Renal dysfunction	K, Ks
Skeletal muscle damage	KYRO, #6

Decreased SGOT	
Hypo function of gonads	F+ or M+
Vitamin B-6 deficiency	B-6

Clinical Nutrition:

For Increased SGOT	For Decreased SGOT
EZV Vitamin E 200	**CTV VITAMIN C THERAPY**
Females: F+	**Females: F+**
Males: M+	**Males: M+**
MIN Multi-Mineral	**MIN Multi-Mineral**
BSV Stress B-Vitamin	*Vitamin B-6*
P Pancreas	*Zinc*
	Manganese

Clinical Crossreference:

- **Asthma** = ↑ SGOT + ↑ HGB (or normal) + ↑ EOS + ↑ LDH + ↑ WBC + ↑ Neut. + ↓ Lymphs. + ↓ Potassium + ↓ Phos. + ↑ Uric Acid
- **Brucellosis** = ↑ SGOT + ↑ Alk Phos. + ↑ WBC + ↑ Lymphs + ↑ Mono. + ↑ Neut. + ↑ SGPT
- **Congestive Heart Failure** = ↑ SGOT + ↑ SGPT + ↑ BUN + ↑ GGTP + ↑ ESR + ↑ MCV + ↑ LDH + ↑ Alk. Phos + ↑ Potassium + ↑ Uric Acid + ↑ Creatinine + ↑ Bilirubin + ↑ Globulin (gamma) + ↑ CO_2 + ↓ Albumin
- **Diabetes** = ↑ SGOT + ↑ Glucose + ↑ Trig. + ↑ LDH
- **Hepatitis** = ↑ SGOT + ↑ SGPT + ↑ GGTP + ↑ Alk. Phos. + ↑ Bilirubin + ↑ Globulin + ↑ Gamma Globulin + ↑ HCT/HGB + ↑ Indirect Bilirubin + WBC's vary with type + ↓ Mag. + ↓ Platlets. Conduct specific hepatitis test.
- **Infection, Actue** = ↑ SGOT + ↑ WBC + ↑ Alk. Phos + ↑ Albumin + ↑ Copper + ↑ ESR + ↑ Globulin + ↓ Iron + ↑ LDH + ↓ Lymphs + ↑ Mono. + ↑ Neut + ↓ Phos. + ↑ BUN + ↑ Uric Acid
- **Influenza** = ↑ SGOT + ↑ Acid. Phos. + ↑ CPK + ↑ ESR + ↓ HCT + Lymphs with decreased T-Lymphs + ↓ Pltelets
- **Mononucleosis** = ↑ SGOT + ↑ SGPT + ↑ GGTP + ↑ Alk. Phos. + ↑ Bilirubin + ↑ Gamma Globulin + ↑ HGB + ↑ LDH + ↑ Mono. + ↑ Neut. + ↑ I_gm + WBC's vary depending on activity of problem. Conduct specific mononucleosis test.
- **Muscular Dystrophy** = ↑ SGOT + ↑ SGPT + ↑ CPK + ↑ LDH + ↓ Creat.
- **Mycardial infarction** = ↑ SGOT + ↑ SGPT + ↑ GGTP + ↑ Acid Phos. + ↑ Alk. Phos + ↑ Chol. + ↑ Creatinine + ↑ ESR + ↑ Glucose + ↑ LDH + ↓ Iron + ↑ WBC + ↑ Trig. + ↑ BUN + ↑ Uric Acid + ↓ Zinc
- **Myocarditis** = ↑ SGOT + ↑ CPK + ↑ LDH + ↑ EOS + ↓ Neut.
- **Oxidation of Orchic Tissue, Decrease (Hypo)** = ↓ SGOT
- **Oxidation of Orchic Tissue, Increase (Hyper)** = ↑ SGOT
- **Pancreatic Dysfunction, Developing** = ↑ SGOT + ↑ LDH + ↓ Cal. + ↓ Triglycerides
- **Parasites** = ↑ SGOT + ↑ EOS + ↑ LDH

- **Rheumatoid Arthritis** = ↓ SGOT (some cases can show ↑ SGOT) + ↑ Alk. Phos + ↓ Alb. ↑ ESR + ↑ Gamma Globulin + ↓ HCT/HGB + ↑ Neut. + ↑ Platlets + ↑ BUN + ↑ Uric Acid

Related Tests:

Acid Phosphatase, Alkaline Phosphatase, CBC, CEA, CPK, PHI, WBC.

Clinical Notes:

- SGOT is usually a more sensitive indicator of chronic tissue damage whereas SGPT is a more sensitive indicator of liver/biliary obstruction.

- Generally, acute viral hepatitis cauese a higher elevation of SGOT than heart attacks.

Practitioner Notes:

- An increased SGOT is generally indicative of liver inflammation, pancreatic inflammation, increased protein synthesis, increased ovary/testicle activity, or heart attack. - J.T.

- A decreased SGOT is generally indicative of reduced protein synthesis, reduced ovary/testicle activity, and reduced enzyme synthesis. - J.T.

Other Notes:

SERUM GLUTAMIC-PYRUVIC TRANSAMINASE (SGPT) also (ALT)

Optimal (Clinical Nutrition) Values: 18 - 22 u/l

Pathological (Lab) Reference Values 2 - 45 u/l

SGPT: Also known as ALT for "Alanine Aminotransferase" is an enzyme present primarily in the liver, and to a lesser extent in the heart, kidneys, and skeletal muscles. It is functionally similar to SGOT with its primary indication to liver. In liver dysfunctions SGPT will remain elevated longer than SGOT and not return to normal as fast. SGPT can help identify dysfunctions in the Reticuloendothelial System (RES), thus it provides insights to the liver (Kupffer cells), spleen, and lymphatic system. Note: Some labs are differentiating between men and women setting the reference values at: Men: 6 - 24 u/l, Women: 4 - 17 u/l.

Pathological Considerations:

Increased SGPT	
Alcoholism	L, Ls, BSV, # 6
Arthritis, Rheumatoid	ARTA, WO SENG, #3
Asthma	R, ACX, Ga
Biliary obstruction	Lb
Brucellosis	GOLD, #3
Choleycystitis	Lb, #3, GOLD
Cirrhosis	L, Ls, OXCC, OXAA, #5
Congestive heart failure	H, Hcv
Dematomyositis	GOLD, TR, XL
Diabetes	P, Ls, L, Gb
Extra-hepatic obstruction	
Free-Radical carcinosis	CTV, OXCC, # 5
Heart disease, ischemic	Hcv, EZV, FLX, MIN
Hepatitis, acute	L, Ls, #4, #3, GOLD
Hepatocellular damage	L, Ls, #5
Hypertension, essential	Ks, HCV
Infections, some	GOLD, #3, VIVI
Influenza	VIVI, ATAK, CDST
Liver dysfunction	L, Ls, #5
Mononucleosis	L, Ls, #4, VIVI
Muscular dystrophy	OXCC, KYRO, #5
Mycardial infarction	H, #6, Hcv
Myocarditis	H, #3, Hcv GOLD, VIVI
Pancreatic dysfunction	P, Ps, #5
Parasites, (occasional)	VRM-1, VRM-3
Renal dysfunction	K, Ks, #5

Decreased SGPT	
No clinical significance	
Liver dysfunction deficiency	L, Ls
Vitamin B-6 Deficiency	BSV

Clinical Nutrition:

For Increased SGPT	
L	Liver
Ls	Liver Stimulant
ACX	Vitamin Detox
LEV	Lecithin

Methionine
Vitamin A
Magnesium

For Decreased SGPT	
LEV	Lecithin
BSV	Stress B Vitamins

Vitamin B-6
Iron
Copper
Methionine

Clinical Crossreference:

- **Alkaline, Over Oxidized, Swollen Liver** = ↑ SGPT
- **Choleycystitis (Bile Duct & Gall Bladder Inflamation)** = ↑ SGPT + ↑ SGOT + ↑ ESR + ↑ WBC + ↑ Neut. + ↑ Alk. Phos. + ↑ Bilirubin + ↓ Platelets + ↓ Albumin + ↓ Total Protein
- **Cirrhosis of the liver** = ↑ SGPT + ↑ SGOT + ↑ GGTP + ↑ TSH + ↑ T-4 + ↑ ESR + ↑ Copper + ↑ Bilirubin + ↑ Globulin + ↑ Alk. Phos. + ↑ Alpha 2 Globulin + ↑ Total Protein + ↓ CAL + ↓ Cholesterol + ↓ RBC + ↓ HCT/HGB + ↓ (NA^+) + ↓ Uric Acid + ↓ Phos. + ↓ Mag. + ↓ Zinc + ↓ Iron + ↓ Albumin
- **Hepatitis** = ↑ SGPT + ↑ SGOT + ↑ GGTP + ↑ Alk. Phos. + ↑ Bilirubin + ↑ Indirect Bilirubin + ↑ Globulin + ↑ Gamma Globulin + ↓ Cholesterol + ↓ HCT/HGB + ↓ Mag.
- **Hypometabolic liver** = ↓ SGPT
- **Liver Disease** = ↑ SGPT + ↑ SGOT + ↑ GGTP + ↑ ESR + ↑ Gamma Globulin + ↑ Alpha 2 Globulin + ↑ LDH + ↑ WBC + ↑ Beta Globulin + ↑ Mag. + ↑ Alk. Phos. + ↑ Bilirubin + ↑ Cholesterol + ↑ Trig. + ↑ Acid Phos. + ↑ Iron + ↓ Albumin + ↓ Alpha 1 Globulin + ↓ BUN + ↓ Blood Platelets, ↓ Protein Bound Iodine + ↓ Zinc
- **Mononucleosis** = ↑ SGPT + ↑ SGOT + ↑ GGTP + ↑ HGB + ↑ IgM + ↑ Mono. + ↑ LDH + ↑ Neut. + ↑ Gamma Globulin + ↑ Alk. Phos. + ↑ Bilirubin

Related Tests:

Alkaline Phosphatase, Bilirubin, Cholesterol, CPK, GGT,, LDH, SGOT.

Clinical Notes:

- SGPT values are greater than SGOT in extra-hepatic obstruction, acute hepatitis and toxic hepatitis. SGOT is greater than SGPT in cirrhosis of the liver, intraheptaic neoplasms and hemolytic jaundice.
- A Vitamin B-6 deficiency causes a decreased SGPT and SGOT.
- Strenuous exercise will not cause an elevation of SGPT, but it does elevate SGOT.

- SGPT is not present in liver cell mitochondria as is SGOT, thus liver cell destruction will elevate SGOT higher than SGOT.

Practitioner Notes:

- SGPT can differentiate jaundice due to liver dysfunction versus hemolytic jaundice. - J.T.
- Increased SGPT is generally indicative of liver or pancreas inflammation or heart attack. - J.T.
- Decreased SGPT is generally indicative of impaired liver function resulting in reduced protein synthesis. - J.T.

Other Notes:

SODIUM (Na^+)

Optimal (Clinical Nutrition) Values: 140 - 144 mEq./l.

Pathological (Lab) Reference Values 135 - 145 mEq./l.

Sodium: (Na^+) Is clinically significant for an understanding of osmolaity and as a pH buffer, and for evaluating adrenal functions, and not for nutritional deficiency or excess. Sodium is the most abundant cat-ion in the extra cellular fluid, but it also plays a critical role inside the cell. It is also involved in the transmission of nerve impulses and functions as a softening agent for tissues. The body closely guards sodium homeostasis via the kidneys and the endocrine system based on the central nervous system's direction. Sodium is a nutrient with a daily requirement of no less than 15 mEq.

Pathological Considerations:

Increased Sodium	
Congestive heart failure	H, Hcv, MIN, EZV
Dehydration	MIN, PTM
Diabetes	P, Ls, L, Gb
Hypercorticadrenalism	Ga, Gb, PTM
Nephritis	K, #3, GOLD
Pyloric obstruction	DCSU, AO, DSIR
Renal dysfunction	K, Ks
Tracheobronchitis	R. GOLD, #3

Decreased Sodium	
Acidosis	Ga, CAL, DIJS
Addison's disease	Ga, #5
Adrenal cortex hypo function	Ga, #1, Gf
Burns	AO, #6, WO
Diabetes	P, Ls, L, Gb
Diarrhea	WO, PTM, GOLD
Edema	Ks, KDIR
Infections, acute	GOLD, #3
Myxedema	Gf, #1, Gb
Nephritis	K, GOLD, #3
Pneumonia	R, #3, #4, GOLD
Pyloric obstruction	DSIR, DCSU
Renal dysfunction	K, Ks, ACX
Sprue	DCSU, D VIVI, ATAK

Clinical Nutrition:

For Increased Chloride

Ks	Kidney Stimulant
K	Kidney

PTM Potassium Stabilizer
Vitamin A

For Decreased Chloride

Ga	Adrenal
K	Kidney

Ks Kidney Stabilizer
DIJS Stomach Antacid
Celery

Clinical Crossreference:

- **Adrenal Cortex Hyperfunction** = ↑ (Na+) + ↓ (K^+) (see Potassium for more values)
- **Adrenal Cortex Hypofunction** = ↓ (Na+) + ↑ (K^+) (see Potassium for more values)
- **Congestive Heart Failure** = ↑ (Na+) + ↑ SGOT + ↑ ALP + ↑ LDH

- **Diabetes** = Altered (Na^+) + ↑ Glucose + ↑ Triglycerides + ↑ LDH
- **Diarrhea** = ↓ (Na^+) + ↑ (K^+)
- **Renal dysfunction** = ↑ (Na^+) + ↑ Creatinine

Related Tests:

Alkaline Phosphatase, BUN, CBC, Cholesterol, HCT, HGB, LDH, SGOT, SGPT, Total Iron, Triglycerides.

Clinical Notes:

- Sodium is an acidifying mineral, antagonistic with Potassium
- There are two forms of Sodium - ionic as in earth and sea salt, and co-valent as is found in vegetables and fruit. Both forms affect the body, but it is the co-valent form that is required by the cells.
- Sodium pumps water and nutrients into the cell
- Sodium is directed by the adrenal cortex hormones.
- Deviations of the sodium balance may occur due to one or more of these conditions:

  1. Excessive or decreased carbonic anhydrase enzyme activity. It controls the rate of sodium excretion by the kidneys.
  2. Increased or decreased blood flow through the kidneys. Increased blood flow causes sodium excretion. Decreased blood flow causes retention.
  3. Increased or decreased renin enzyme activity. Renin increases aldosterone secretion and regulates the blood flow to the kidneys. Increased or decreased blood flow alters sodium levels. The most common effect of renin is its increased presence which leads to water retention an hypertension.
  4. Aldosterone, an adrenal hormone, acts on the distal tubules and is responsive to renin, ACTH, sodium levels, and potassium levels. If excessive, sodium will be retained, leading to hypertension.
  5. Steroidal hormones such as estrogen and progesterone controlled by the anterior pituitary affect sodium levels and an imbalance in these hormones can cause pre-menstrual water retention.
  6. Vassopressin, the anti diuretic hormone, controls water re absorption via the kidneys, distal tubules, and thus sodium.

Warning:

- Sodium less than 120 mEq/l is indicative of severe, emergency electrolyte imbalance.
- Sodium greater than 155 mEq/l is indicative of severe, emergency electrolyte imbalance.

Practitioner Notes:

- Consider salt intake and perspiration. Lack of salt or frequent, heavy perspiration can induce low serum sodium levels. Most people can do a perspiration taste test to determine if they have adequate salt levels. Taste your perspiration from an outer shoulder away from face or hair. If there is only a slight saline taste, the level of salt is usually adequate. - R.M.

- Low sodium values are usually more reflective of excessive water in the body rather than a sodium deficiency. - J.T.

Other Notes:

TRI-IODOTHYRONINE UPTAKE, (T3 UPTAKE)

Optimal (Clinical Nutrition) Values 26 - 30

Pathological (Lab) Reference Values: 23 - 33%

T3 Uptake: Is a measurement of tri-iodothyronine uptake by a treated resin which determines the degree of saturation of the thyroid binding Globulin. This is not the bloodstream's T3 level. Before T3 is released into the bloodstream, thyroglobulin is taken up by the thyroid's follicular cells and converted by proteolytic enzymes to T3 and T4. The "3" in T3 refers to the number of iodine atoms joined to a thyroglobin molecule. T3 is four times more potent than T4 (Thyroxine) in its metabolic action. Note: T3 RIA is a different test of T3 that measures the total T3 hormone in circulation by Radio Immuno Assay. It provides a more accurate insight of thyroid status.

Pathological Considerations:

Increased T3 Uptake	
Graves Disease	Gf, #5, Gb, FLX
Hyperthyroidism	Gf, Gb, FLX
Protein Malnutrition	PRO, D
Renal Dysfunction	K, Ks, Gf
Thyroxine (Armor) Therapy	Gf

Decreased T3 Uptake	
Estrogen Drug Therapy	Ft, Gf
Hypothyroidism	Gf, #1, Gb
Pregnancy	Gf
Thyroid Drug Therapies	Gf

Clinical Nutrition:

For Increased T3 Uptake	
Gf	Thyroid
Gb	Pituitary

For Decreased T3 Uptake	
Gf	Thyroid
#1	Activator
Gb	Pituitary

Clinical Crossreference:

- **Estrogen Drug Therapy** = ↓ T3 + ↑ T4 + ↑ TBG (Thyroid Binding Globulin)
- **Hyperthyroidism** = ↑ T3 Uptake + ↑ T4 + ↑ BUN + ↑ EOS + ↑ Gastrin + ↑ Glucose + ↑ Alk. Phos. + ↑ Phos. + ↓ Baso + ↓ Albumin + ↓ Calcium + ↓ HCT + ↓ HGB + ↓ MCV + ↓ Magnesium + ↓ Total Protein + ↓ Plasma Renin + ↓ Cholesterol + ↓ Triglycerides
- **Hypothyroidism** = ↓ T3 Uptake + ↓ T4 + ↓ Alk. Phos + ↓ Gastein + ↓ HCT + ↓ HGB + ↓ Iron + ↓ Sodium + ↑ Albumin + ↑ Calcium + ↑ LDH + ↑ Magnesium + ↑ Baso + ↑ Cholesterol + ↑ Trig.
- **Protein Malnutrition** = ↑ T3 + ↓ Total Protein (See Total Protein)
- **Renal Dysfunction** = ↑ T3 Uptake + ↑ Creatinine (See Creatinine)

Related Tests:

Protein Bound Iodine, TSH, T3, T4, T7.

Clinical Notes:

- In Grave's disease, the pituitary's TSH (Thyroid Stimulating Hormone) is decreased in plasma in its hyperthyroid stage; at normal range in the Grave's euthyroid stage, and increased if the thyroid becomes unresponsive or hypo.
- TSH is elevated in hypothyroidism unless the low thyroid function is due to an anterior pituitary hypofunction.
- Decreased T3 Uptake is helpful to ascertain hyperthyroidism.
- Altered T3 Uptake provides insights to the thyroid's functional abilities, but does not reveal the cause of dysfunction.

Practitioner Notes:

- Thyroid nutritional supplementation is beneficial for people on drug-thyroxine such as Synthroid® or Armor® thyroid because thyroxine replacement only accounts for one of several thyroid hormones. - J.T.
- Thyroxine medication causes atrophy of the thyroid. Nutrition and therapeutic supplements can help avoid addiction to thyroid medications if the medications haven't been used o the point of thyroid atrophy. - J.T.

Other Notes:

TETRA-IODOTHYRONINE (T4)

Optimal (Clinical Nutrition) Values 7 - 8.5

Pathological (Lab) Reference Values: 5.0 - 13.4

T4: Refers to Thyroxine, one of the thyrod gland's hormones, and chief regulator of metabolic activity throughout the body. Thyroxine is secreted after thyroglobin is taken up by the follicular cells in a process involving several enzymes. Malfunction in this series of reactions can cause hypothyroidism and goitre swellings. In T4, the "4" refers to the number of Iodine atoms joined to the thyroglobulin molecule by tyrosine. The pituitary's thyroid stimulating hormone governs the rate at which the thyroid produces and secretes thyroxine. The liver breaks down thyroxine which is then excreted in the bile as inorganic iodine.

T4, along with T3, functions to increase the rate of metabolic activity, maintain body temperature, regulate carbohydrate/fat/protein catbolism in the cells, maintain growth hormone release, contol skeletal muscle maturation, and regulate the heart rate and its force and output. It promotes central nervous system growth, helps maintain muscle tone, and stimulates tissues to synthesize hormones.

Pathological Considerations:

Increased T4	
Adrenal fatigue	Ga, #6
Anovulatory Drugs	F+, Gf
Cirrhosis	L, Ls, OXAA, OXCC, #6
Drug addiction	Gf, Ga, ACX
Early Hepatitis	L, Ls, GOLD, VIVI
Hyperthyroidism	Gf, Gb, #6, #5
Pregnancy	Gf
Thyrotoxicosis	Gf, Gb #5

Decreased T4	
Adrenal hyperfunction	Ga, #5
Cretinism	B, I, Gb, Gf
Diabetes	Gb, L, Ls, P
Hypoproteinemia	PRO, D, Gf
Hypothyroidism	Gf, #1, Gb
Myxedema	Gf, #1
Nephrosis	K, Ks
Pituitary, Anterior hypofunction	Gb, #1
Renal Dysfunction	K, Ks
Simmonds Disease	Gb, #1

Clinical Nutrition:

For Increased T4

Gf	**Thyroid**
L	**Liver**
CAL	**Calcium Plus**

Iodine
Vitamin D

For Decreased T4

Gf	**Thyroid**
Gb	**Pituitary**
#1	**Activator**

L Liver
LEV Lecithin
Vitamin B-6
Magnesium
Kelp
Dulse

Clinical Crossreference:

- **Hypermetabolic Thyroid** = ↑ T3 + ↑ T4 + ↑ T7 (See T3 Uptake)
- **Hypometabolic Thyroid** = ↓ T3 + ↓ T4 + ↓ T 7

- **Diabetes** = ↓ T4 + ↑ Glucose (See Glucose)
- **Protein Malnutrition** = ↓ T4 + ↓ Total Protein (See Protein, Total)
- **Renal Dysfunction** = ↓ T4 + ↑ Creat. (See Creatinine)

Related Tests:

Protein Bound Iodine (PBI), T3 RIA, T3 Uptake, T7, TAT (Thyroid Autoantibody Test), TBG, TSH.

Clinical Notes:

- Hypothyroidism - the most useful tests to determine if hypothyroidism is a concern are T-4, FTI, and TSH.
- Hyperthyroidism - the most useful tests to determine if hyperthyroidism is a concern are T-4, FTI, and Total T-3.
- Average 80 - 220 NG/DL - Triiodothyronine by radioimmunoassay is used to confirm or rule out suspected hyperthyroidism when T3, T4 and T7 are essentially normal and clinical signs strongly suggest hyperthyroidism.
- Many clinicians recommend the same therapy for high or low T4 values: such therapies assist the thyroid to balance regardless of the deviation.
- Altered bilirubin may give false T4 values.

Practitioner Notes:

- Administration of synthetic thyroxine can cause atrophy of the thyroid and dependency on the drug therapy. With continued use of thyroid medication, can cause a suppression of thyrotropin (TSH) secretion by the pituitary contributing to further thyroid inactivity and dependence on medication. - J.T.
- The thyroid makes several hormones, yet Medicine traditionally prescribes only thyroxine. If thyroxine therapy causes atrophy or suppressed thyroid function, other metabolic problems can develop particularly with the endocrine feed-back loops involving the adrenals and the gonads, as well as with calcium metabolism. - J.T.
- Increased T-4 is indicative of the endocrine feedback loop of hyper thyroid, hyper adrenal, and hyper gonads, and hypo anterior pituitary. - J.T.
- Decreased T-4 is indicative of the endocrine feedback loop of hypo thyroid, hyper adrenal, hypo gonads, and hyper anterior pituitary. - J.T.

Other Notes:

T7, FREE THYROXINE INDEX (FTI)

Optimal (Clinical Nutrition) Values 1.9 - 2.5

Pathological (Lab) Reference Values: 1.0 - 4.0

T7: Is a calculation obtained by multiplying T3 Uptake times T4. (T3 ÷ 100) X T4 = T7. The value of this test is based on the concept that T3 Uptake is inversely proportional to serum Unsaturated Thyroid Binding Globulin (UTBG), and that free T4 varies directly with Total T4 but inversely to UTBG. There is a noteworthy margin of error in using T7 diagnostically in that occasionally in patients on hormones, a normal T7 can be calculated when there is an abnormal T3, or T4. T7 provides insights into the metabolic impact of thyroid hormone.

Pathological Considerations:

Increased T7		Decreased T7	
Hyperthyroidism	Gf, #6, Gb	Hypothyroidism	Gf, #1, Gb

Clinical Nutrition:

For Increased T7	For Decreased T7
Gf Thyroid	**Gf Thyroid**
Gb Pituitary	**Gb Pituitary**
#6 Healer	**#1 Activator**
L Liver	L Liver
CAL CAlcium Plus	LEV Lecithin
Iodine	*B-6*
Vitamin D	*Kelp/Dulse*
	Magnesium

Clinical Crossreference:

- **Hypermetabolic Thyroid** = ↑ T3 + ↑ T4 + ↑ T7 (See T3 Uptake)
- **Hypometabolic Thyroid** = ↓ T3 + ↓ T4 + ↓ T7 (See T3 Uptake)

Related Tests:

TBG, TSH, T3 Uptake, T4.

Clinical Notes:

- Average 80 - 220 NG/DL - Triiodothyronine by radioimmunoassay is used to confirm or rule out suspected hyperthyroidism when T3, T4 and T7 are essentially normal and clinical signs strongly suggest hyperthyroidism.
- People with low thyroid values are often advised to avoid soybeans, rutabaga, brussel sprouts, cabbage, kale, cauliflower and kohlrabi until their values are normal.
- Many practitioners recommend the same therapy for high and low values.

Practitioner Notes:

Other Notes:

TRIGLYCERIDES

Optimal (Clinical Nutrition) Values 80 - 115 mg/dl.

Pathological (Lab) Reference Values: 30 - 200 mg/dl.

Triglycerides: Are blood fats consisting of glycerol esterified with three fatty acids (CHO + fatty acids). They are fundamentally manufactured in the liver from fatty acids, but can be derived directly from excess glucose. Thus excessive refined carbohydrate (sugar) intake is a major cause of elevated triglycerides. Cholesterol and triglycerides travel in the bloodstream together, so triglycerides are included in cardiovascular profiles. Triglycerides are an important source of energy at the cellular level. The triglyceride test reveals potential atherosclerosis and fat metabolism problems.

Pathological Considerations:

Increased Triglycerides	
Alcoholism	AZV, MIN, L, #5
Arteriosclerosis	HCV, FLX, EZV, MIN
Atherosclerosis	HCV, FLX, EZV, MIN
B-12 Anemia	BSV, MIN
Cardiac Stress	H, CAL, FLX. Hcv
Coronary Artery Disease	HCV
Diabetes	P, L, Gb, Ls
Glycogen storage disease	L Ls
Gout	K, PTM, Ls
Hepatitis	L, Ls, Gold
Hyperlipidism	D, Ls
Hypothyroidism	Gf, #1, Gb, L
Liver dysfunction	L, Ls, #5
Myocardial infarction	H, #6, Hcv
Pancreas dysfunction	P, Ps, #5
Pregnancy	L,
Renal dysfunction	K, Ks, #5
Respiratory dysfunction]	R, ACX, Hcv

Decreased Triglycerides	
Brain infarction	B, Hcv, #6
Hyperparathyroidism	Gf, Cal
Hyperthyroidism	Gf Gb
Hypochlorhydria	D, #1
Liver congestion	LEV, Ls
Mal-nourishment	PRO, AZV, MIN

Clinical Nutrition:

For Increased Triglycerides

FLX	Flax Seed Oil
B	Brain
Gb	Pituitary
Lb	Liver Normalizer
Hcv	Cardiovascular

Low fat, no refined carbohydrates with complex carbohydrate diet and limited fruits and juices. Fresh fruit is o.k. but not bottled juices. (See Pro-Vita! Plan)

Gf Thyroid

(contiued)

For Decreased Triglycerides

LEV	Lecithin
FLX	Vdg. Omega-3 Flax Seed
Gb	Pituitary

B Brain

Ps Pancreas Stabilizer

LEV Lecithin
BSV Stress B-Vitamin
Ps Pancreas Stabilizer
Carnitine
Chromium picolinate
Zinc
Magnesium Orotate
STOP ALCOHOL
STOP SUGAR

Clinical Crossreference:

- **Alcoholism** = ↑ Triglycerides + ↑ GGTP (See GGTP)
- **Arteriosclerosis** = ↑ Triglycerides + ↑ Uric Acid + ↑ Cholesterol (See Cholesterol)
- **Cardiac Stress** = ↑ Triglycerides + ↑ SGOT (See SGOT)
- **Diabetes Mellitus, Tendency** = ↑ Triglycerides + ↑ LDH + ↑ Glucose
- **Gout** = ↑ Triglycerides + ↑ Uric Acid (See Uric Acid)
- **Hepatitis** = ↑ Triglycerides + ↑ SGPT (See SGPT)
- **Hypochlorhydria** = ↓ Triglycerides + ↑ Globulin (See Globulin, Total)
- **Lipase & Chromium, Need For** = ↓ Triglycerides + ↓ Calcium + ↑ LDH
- **Liver Dysfunction** = ↑ Triglycerides + ↑ GGTP + ↑ SGPT (See SGPT)
- **Malnutrition** = ↓ Triglycerides + ↓ Total Protein (See Protein, Total)
- **Pancreas Dysfunction** = ↑ Triglycerides + Altered Glucose (See Glucose)
- **Respiratory Distress** = ↑ Triglycerides + ↓ Total Protein (See Protein, Total)

Related Tests:

Amylase, BUN, CPK, Creatinine, GGT, Glycohemoglobin, LDH, SGOT, SGPT, T3, T4, TSH.

Clinical Notes:

- For an accurate test, the patient must be fasting (12 hours) and abstaining fro alcohol (24 hours).
- Elevated triglycerides without elevated cholesterol is not indicative of potential heart disease.
- Triglycerides are influenced by the nervous system and can elevated when a person is under stress.
- Birth control pills cause Triglycerides to elevate.

Practitioner Notes:

- For sedentary people with elevated Triglycerides, exercise will reduce levels. - J.T.
- Low thyroid function results in elevated triglycerides. Consider thyroid supplementation to correct this. - J.T.

Other Notes:

URIC ACID

Optimal (Clinical Nutrition) Values: 4.5 - 5.5

Pathological (Lab) Reference Values 2.2 - 9.9
Male 3.9 - 9.0/Female 2.2 - 3.3

Uric Acid: Is an end result of cells being broken down in the body. Its level also reflects the consumption of purine rich foods like sweet breads, liver, and kidneys. High levels of uric acid can be a warning sign before gout.

Pathological Considerations:

Increased Uric Acid

RENAL INSUFFICIENCY

Acute & chronic nephritis	K, #3, Gold
Increased poisoning, e.g. mercury and lead	CLNZ, CTV, ACX
Hypertension	HCV

METABOLIC DISTURBANCES

Arthritis, rhematoid	ARTA, SENG, #3
Diabetes with acidosis	P, Ls, L, Gb
Exercise, strenuous	
Gout	K
Purines, excessive in diet	Reduce

CONDITIONS WITH DESTRUCTION OF CELL NUCLEI

Leukemia	OXCC, OXAA, #5, S
Malignant tumers	OXCC, #5, OXAA
Pernicious or any severe anemia	BLDB, MIN
Polycythemia	OXAA, BLDB, #5

MISCELLANEOUS

Acute infections	GOLD, #3
Arteriosclerosis	Hcv, D, MIN
Asthma	R, Ga, ACX
Cardiac decompensation	H
Eclampsia	N-3, Nc
Folic Acid deficiency	BSV, AZV
Free_Radical Pathologrs	CLNZ, CTV, EZV, OXOX
Hyperparathyroidism	Gf, Gb
Intestinal obstruction	C
Liver dysfunction	L, Ls
Prostetic obstruction	KDIR, Mpc
Thymus dysfunction	Gt
Urinary obstruction	KDIR

Decreased Uric Acid

Acute yellow atrophy of the liver	L, Ls, Lb
Liver dysfunction (cirrhosis)	OXCC, Ls, L, Lb
Pernicious anemia--relapse	BLDB, BSV, MIN
Pregnancy	L, ACP
Salcylate and atrophine therapy	ACX

Clinical Nutrition:

For Increased Uric Acid	
Gt	Thymus
Ps	Pancreas Stimulant
BSV	Stress B-Vitamin

Magnesium
Folic Acid (Folate)

For Decreased Uric Acid	
P	Pancreas
D	Digestive

Clinical Crossreference:

- **Pancreatic Dnzyme Deficiency** = ↑ Uric Acid + ↑ Protein + Altered Calcium
- **Thymus Dysfunction** = ↑ Uric Acid + ↑ Bilirubin
- **Potential Heart Attack** = ↑ Glucose + ↑ Cholesterol + ↑ Triglycerides + ↑ Uric Acid
- **Chymotryspin Deficiency** = ↓ Uric Acid + ↑ Cholesterol + ↑ Triglycerides
- **Excessive Tissue Fluid** = ↓ Uric Acid + ↓ B U N

Related Tests:

Alk. Phos., HGB, GGTP, LDH, SGOT, SGPT.

Clinical Notes:

Practitioner Notes:

- After hepatitis, chemotherapy, or other liver stress, folate conversion through the five steps of hepatic processing may be permanently impaired. Here the 5 formyl-tetrahydrafolate converted in the intestine by heat to the 5 methyl-tetrahydrafolate form that is immediately available to the cell can offer a simple solution. - R.M.
- Increased Uric Acid is generally indicative of increased nucleo protein utilization, high protein diets, and metabolic acidosis. - J.T.
- Decreased Uric Acid is generally indicative of reduced nucleic acid utilization or an overactive anterior pituitary. - J.T.

Other Notes:

WHITE BLOOD COUNT, TOTAL (WBC)

Optimal (Clinical Nutrition) Values 5,000 - 7,000 k/cu.mm.

Pathological (Lab) Reference Values: 4 - 11 k/cu.mm.

WBC: White Blood Cells (leukocytes) are the immune system's infection fighting cells. In a healthy individual there is normally one WBC to every 500 red blood cells (RBC). If a bacterial infection occurs, the WBC count increases substantially. If a viral infection occurs, the WBC may or may not increase depending on how the immune system responds.

There are two categories of WBCs each with specialized cells: 1) Granulocytes including neutrophils (polymorphonucleocytes called "polys", "stabs" which are immature neutrophils), Basophils (BASO), and Eosinophils (EOS); and 2) Non-granulocytes including Lymphocytes (lymphs), and Monocytes (Monos). The WBC is the total of all these cells. A differential test is run to count the individual types of cells making up the total, providing further insight into the cause of any altered count.

Pathological Considerations:

Increased WBC	
Abcesses	GOLD, WO
Adrenal Dysfunction	Ga
Asthma	R, Ga, ACX
Emphysema	R, #5
Flu with Bacterial Infection	VIVI, GOLD, ACX
Free Radical Pathologies	OXCC, #5, CTV
Infections (bacterial)	GOLD, #3
Leukemia	OXCC, S, #5
Measles	VIVI, GOLD, ACX
Mononucleosis (days 7 - 21)	L, Ls, GOLD, VIVI
Mumps	VIVI, ACX
Parasites	VRM-1, VRM-3
Whooping Cough	R, GOLD, VIVI, S

Decreased WBC	
Adrenal dysfunction	Ga
Anemias (B-Vitamin)	BSV
Bone Marrow, Depression	BLDB, OXAA
Chicken pox	VIVI, ACX
Chronic Infection	ATAK, OXOX, #3
Flu, early stage	VIVI, CDST, ACX
Free radical pathologies	OXCC, #5, CTV
Hepatitis	L, Ls, GOLD
Hyperparathyroidism	Gf
Leukemia, Aleukemic	OXCC, S, #5
Lupus, syst. eryth	OXCC, OXAA, S, #5
Measles, late	VIVI, GOLD, ACX
Mononucleosis (days 1 - 7)	L, Ls, GOLD, VIVI
Parasites, chronic	VRM-1, VRM-3
Pituitary, anterior dysfunction	Gb
Rheumatoid Arthritis	ARTA, SENG, #3
Rubella, prior to rash	VIVI, ACX VIVI

Clinical Nutrition:

For Increased WBC	
Gf	Thymus
S	Spleen
CTV	Vitamin C Therapy
PRO	Nutro Protein
LEV	Lecithin
ACX	Vitamin Detox
Zinc	

For Decreased WBC	
LEV	LECITHIN
PRO	Nutro-Protein
Gt	Thymus
CTV	Vitamin C therapy
Zinc	
Vitamin A	

Clinical Crossreference:

- **Adrenal Dysfunction** = Alt. WBC + Alt. Potassium (See Potassium)
- **Anemia, B-Vitamin** = ↓ WBC + Alt. MCV/MCH (See MCV)
- **Asthma** = ↑ WBC + ↑ HGB (See HGB)
- **Chicken Pox** = ↑ WBC + ↑ Alb. + ↑ HCT + ↑ Lymphs + ↑ Neut. + ↑ BASO + ↑ HGB + ↑ Bilirubin + ↑ Gamma Globulin
- **Flu** = Alt. WBC + ↑ ESR + ↑ CPK + ↑ SGOT + ↑ Lymph + ↑ Acid Phos. + ↓ HCT + ↓ Platelets + ↓ T-Lymphs
- **Infection, Acute** = ↑ WBC + ↑ Neut. + ↑ Copper + ↑ Alk. Phos + ↑ Uric Acid + ↑ Monos + ↑ BUN + ↑ LDH + ↑ ESR + ↓ Lymphs Alb. + ↓ Phos. + ↓ Iron
- **Infection, Chronic** = ↓ WBC + ↓ Neut. + ↓ Iron + ↓ HCT/HGB + ↑ ESR + ↑ Glob. + ↑ Copper + ↑ BASO + Alt. Lymphs
- **Lupus** = ↓ WBC + ↓ Alb. + ↓ Platelets + ↓ Lymphs + ↓ HCT/HGB + ↑ ESR + ↑ LDH + ↑ SGPT + ↑ I_gA, D, H, M + ↑ Copper + ↑ Alpha 1 & 2 + ↑ Gamma Glob.
- **Measles** = Alt. WBC + ↑ Bilirubin + ↓ HCT + ↓ Lymph + ↓ Neut.
- **Mumphs** = ↑ WBC + ↑ Monos + ↑ ESR + ↓ Glucose + ↓ Alb.
- **Parasites** = Alt. WBC + ↑ EOS (See EOS)
- **Rubella** = ↓ WBC + ↓ Neut. + ↓ Platlets + ↑ Lymphs
- **Whopping Cough (Pertussis)** = ↑ WBC + ↑ Lymphs + ↓ Neut.

Related Tests:

- Baso, EOS, Lymphs, Monos, Neut.

Clinical Notes:

- Many drugs interfere with the body's natural response and can alter, derange and suppress the immune system. Drugs designed to stop the immune system's natural processes include: antibiotics, aspirin, ibuprofen, acetaminophen and cortisone. Such interference with the immune system is suspected to be linked as one of several causes of auto immune disorders.

- WBCs can vary as much as 2 k/cu.mm a day as a result of exercise, saunas, smoking, stress, diet and minor infections.

UNFAVORABLE SIGNS

- Extreme leukocytosis with high percentage of neutrophils.
- Failure to develop leukocytosis.
- High proportion of immature neutrophils (stabs).
- Numerous toxic forms.
- Marked absolute reduction of lymphocytes.

BLOOD PICTURE DURING RECOVERY

- Decrease in total leukocyte count and neutrophils.
- Decrease of immature forms.
- Temporary increase of monocytes.
- Increase of eosinophiols.
- Increase of lymphocytes.
- Absence or decrease of toxic forms.
- Women over 40 years of age tend to have low WBCs.
- A low WBC with a low lymph count (below 19) is often indicative of carcinoid free radical pathology.

Practitioner Notes:

- Diets based on vegetables and the Pro-Vita! Plan help keep WBCs in the low-optimal range. Diets based on cooked foods and animal protein tend to elevate WBCs as they are perpetually occupies with the excessive "dead food". - J. T.

- Excessive doses of Ascorbic Acid (Vitamin C) can inhibit the histamine response, and thus inhibit the macrophage response to the site of inflammation. This is an example where excessive vitamin therapy can be suppressive to overall health. - J. T.

Other Notes:

Index To Health Conditions & Confirmatory Blood Tests

ACIDOSIS

INCREASE	DECREASE
Chlor	Calcium
K^+	CO_2

ADRENAL CORTEX HYPERFUNCTION

INCREASE	DECREASE
Na^+	K^+
Chlor	Renin
Cortisol	
Aldosterone	
CO_2	

ADRENAL CORTEX HYPOFUNCTION

INCREASE	DECREASE
K^+	Chlor
Renin	Na^+
	Cortisol
	Aldesterone
	CO_2

ADRENAL DYSFUNCTION

INCREASE	DECREASE
Neut	
Alt K^+	

ADRENAL HYPERFUNCTION

INCREASE	DECREASE
K^+	Protein

ADRENAL HYPOFUNCTION

INCREASE	DECREASE
Protein	K^+

ALB. DEPRESSED DUE TO LIVER DYSFUNCTION

INCREASE	DECREASE
Alt. SGPT	Albumin
Alt. GGT	

ALCOHOLISM

INCREASE	DECREASE
GGTP	K+
SGPT	Plasma Phos.
SGOT	Platlets
Alk. Phos.	
Cal	
Copper	
Bilirubin	
CPK	
FSH	
LDH	
PTH	
Plasma	
Cort.	
Serum Phos.	
Trig.	
Uric Acid	

ALKALOSIS

INCREASE	DECREASE
CO_2	Cal.
	Chlor.
	K^+
	BUN

ANEMIA, IRON DEFICIENCY

INCREASE	DECREASE
	Iron
	MCV
	MCHC

ANEMIA, PERNICIOUS, VITAMIN B-12

INCREASE	DECREASE
MCV	Alb.
MCH	RBC
EPS	Chol.
LDH	HCT
Ind. Bili.	HGB
Gastrin	K^+
Copper	B-12
	Folate
	Uric Acid

ANEMIA, FOLIC ACID

INCREASE	DECREASE
MCV	Alk. Phos.
MCH	K^+
Iron	Folate
LDH	Uric Acid
Copper	Platlets
Lymph	RBC
Bili.	HGB
	HCT
	Neut.

ANEMIA, VITAMIN B-6

INCREASE	DECREASE
HGB	MCV
Mono.	MCH
Iron	HCT
	WBC
	Neut

ANEMIA, IRON

INCREASE	DECREASE
	MCV
	HGB

ANTERIOR PITUITARY DYSFUNCTION

INCREASE	DECREASE
Cal.	Cort.
Chol.	FSH
EOS	HCT
	HGB
	HGH
	Lutenizing hormone
	Plasma Aldesterone
	Plasma Progesterone
	Plasma Testosterone

ARTERIOSCLEROSIS

INCREASE	DECREASE
Chol.	HDL
BUN	
CO2	
LDH (VLDL)	
Copper	
Uric Acid	
Creat.	
Trig.	

ARTHRITIS

INCREASE	DECREASE
SGOT	ALP
Uric Acid	Alb.
	Lymphs
	Copper
	Gamma Glob.
	Neut.
	Platlets

ASTHMA

INCREASE	DECREASE
SGOT	Lymphs
HGB	K^+
EOS	Phos.
LDH	Uric Acid
WBC	
Neut.	

BILIARY OBSTRUCTION

INCREASE	DECREASE
GGTP	Vitamin K
SGPT	
SGOT	
Acid Phos.	
Trig.	
Amylase	
Bili.	
Chol.	
Globulin (Alpha 2, Beta)	
WBC	
LDH	
Vitamin A	

BRUCELLOSIS

INCREASE	DECREASE
SGOT	
Alk. Phos.	
WBC	
Lymphs	
Mono.	
Neut.	
SGPT	

CADMIUM HEAVY METAL TOXICITY

INCREASE	DECREASE
Calcium	Phos.
	Urinary Phos.
	MCV

CARDIAC DYSFUNCTION

INCREASE	DECREASE
LDH	
SGOT	
Chol	

CHICKEN POX

INCREASE	DECREASE
WBC	
Alb.	
HCT	
Lymphs	
Neut.	
Baso.	
HGB	
Bili.	
Gamma Globulin	

CHOLEYCYSTITIS

INCREASE	DECREASE
SGPT	Platlets
SGOT	Alb.
ESR	Total Protein
WBC	
Neut.	
Neut.	
Alk. Phos.	
Bili.	

CHYMOTRYpsIN DEFICIENCY

INCREASE	DECREASE
Chol.	Uric Acid
Trig.	

CIRRHOSIS OF THE LIVER

INCREASE	DECREASE
SGPT	Calcium
SGOT	Chol.
GGTP	RBC
TSH	HCT/HGB
T4	NA^+
ESR	Uric Acid
Copper	Phos.
Bili.	Mag.
Glob.	Zinc
Alk. Phos.	Iron
Alpha 2 Glob.	Alb.
Total Protein	

CO_2 DEFICIENT

INCREASE	DECREASE
Chlor.	Calcium
K^+	CO_2

CO_2 EXCESS

INCREASE	DECREASE
CO_2	Cal.
BUN	K^+

CONGESTIVE HEART FAILURE

INCREASE	DECREASE
SGOT	Alb.
SGPT	
BUN	
GGTP	
ESR	
MCV	
LDH	
Alk. Phos.	
K+	
Uric Acid	
Creat.	
Bili.	
Globulin	
CO2	

DERMATOMYOSITIS

INCREASE	DECREASE
EOS	HGB
Alpha 2 Glob.	
ESR	
LDH	
Gamma. Glob.	
WBC	
HCT	
EOS	
LDH	

DIABETES

INCREASE	DECREASE
Glucose	
Trig.	
LDH	
SGOT	
Creat.	
BUN	
Chol.	
Uric Acid	
Acid Phos.	

DIGESTIVE HYPOCHLORHYDRIA

INCREASE	DECREASE
Glob.	CO2
Alk. Phos.	Alb.
	Calcium
	Phos.
	B-12
	Folates
	Parathyroid Hormone

DIGESTIVE INFLAMATION

INCREASE	DECREASE
MCH	Total Protein
Uric Acid	Alb.
Baso	HCT/HGB
EOS	Lymphs
Gamma Iso-Fraction	B-12
Polyps	Cal.
	Glob.
	Sodium
	K^+
	MCH
	MCHC

EDEMA IN EXTREMITIES

INCREASE	DECREASE
	Alb.
	Total Protein

EMPHYSEMA

INCREASE	DECREASE
HGB	Phos.
HCT	Chlor.
K^+	Alpha
Amonia	Alpha Antitrypsin
CO_2	

FAT ABSORPTION, POOR

INCREASE	DECREASE
	Phos.
	Cal.
	Bili.

FATTY LIVER CONGESTION

INCREASE	DECREASE
	GGTP
	SGPT
	Chol.

FLU

INCREASE	DECREASE
Alb. WBC	HCT
ESR	Platlets
CPK	T-Lymphs
SGOT	
Lymph	
Acid Phos.	

FOOD ALLERGIES

INCREASE	DECREASE
EOS	
IgE	

GASTRITIS/COLITIS

INCREASE	DECREASE
MCV	Alb.
Uric Acid	Total Protein
Baso	HCT/HGB
EOS	Lymphs
Gamma	B-12
Iso-Fraction	Cal.
Polys	Glob.
	Sodium
	K+
	MCH
	MCHC

GOUT

INCREASE	DECREASE
Creat.	
Uric Acid	
Trig.	

HEPATITIS

INCREASE	DECREASE
SGOT	Mag.
SGPT	Platlets
GGTP	WBC's vary with type
Alk. Phos.	
Bili.	
Glob.	
Gamma Glob.	
HCT/HGB	
Indirect Bili.	

HYPER-CORTICOADRENALISM

INCREASE	DECREASE
Cort.	K^+
Chlor.	Renin
Na^+	
CO	

HYPER-PARATHYROIDISM

INCREASE	DECREASE
PTH	Phos.
Cal.	Trig.
Uric Acid	Chol..
Creat.	Mag.
Gastrin	
CO2	
Alk. Phos.	
Chlor.	
Acid Phos.	

HYPERTHYROIDISM

INCREASE	DECREASE
T3 Uptake	Baso
T4	Alb.
BUN	Cal.
EOS	HCT/HGB
Gastrin	MCV
Glucose	Mag.
Alk. Phos.	
Phos.	

HYPOPARATHYROID

INCREASE	DECREASE
Phos.	PTH
Uric Acid	Alk. Phos.
	Cal.

IMMUNODEFICIENCY

INCREASE	DECREASE
MCV	Gamma Glob.
	Alb.
	HCT
	HGB
	Total Protein
	WBC
	Platlets
	Lymphs

INFECTION, ACUTE

INCREASE	DECREASE
SGOT	Iron
WBC	Lymphs
Alk. Phos.	Phos.
Alb.	
Copper	
ESR	
Glob.	
LDH	
Mono.	
Neut.	
BUN	
Uric Acid	

INFECTION, CHRONIC

INCREASE	DECREASE
ESR	WBC
Glob	Neut.
Copper	Iron
Baso	HCT/HGB
Lymphs	

IRON DEFICIENCY

INCREASE	DECREASE
Bili.	HGB
Glob.	HCT
B-12	Iron
	MCV
	MCHC

LIVER DISEASE

INCREASE	DECREASE
SGPT	Alb.
SGOT	Alpha 1 Glob.
GGTP	BUN
ESR	Blood Platlets
Gamma Glob.	Protein Bound Iodine
Alpha 2 Glob.	Zinc
LDH	
WBC	
Beta Glob.	
Mag.	
Alk. Phos.	
Bili.	
Chol.	
Trig.	
Acid. Phos.	
Iron	

LUPUS

INCREASE	DECREASE
ESR	WBC
LDH	Alb.
SGPT	Platlets
IgA, D, H, M	Lymphs
Copper	HCT/HGB
Alpha 1 & 2	
Gamma Glob.	

MEASLES

INCREASE	DECREASE
Alt. WBC	HCT
Bilirubin	Lymphs
	Neut.

MONONUCLEOSIS

INCREASE	DECREASE
SGOT	
SGPT	
GGTP	
Alk. Phos.	
Bili.	
Gamma Glob.	
HGB	
LDH	
Mono.	
Neut.	
I_gE	

MULTIPLE SCLEROSIS

INCREASE	DECREASE
Chol.	Phospholipids
IgE	Vitamin B-12
GGTP	Lymphs
Alpha 1 & 2	
Alb.	
Beta Gamma Glob.	

MUMPHS

INCREASE	DECREASE
WBC	Glucose
Monos	Alb.
ESR	

MUSCULAR DYSTROPHY

INCREASE	DECREASE
SGOT	Creat.
SGPT	
CPK	
LDH	

MYCARDIAL INFECTION

INCREASE	DECREASE
SGOT	Iron
SGPT	Zinc
GGTP	
Acid Phos.	
Alk. Phos.	
Chol.	
Creat.	
ESR	
Glucose	
LDH	
WBC	
Trig	
BUN	
Uric Acid	

MYOCARDITIS

INCREASE	DECREASE
SGOT	Neut.
CPK	
LDH	
EOS	

OSTEOPOROSIS

INCREASE	DECREASE
Alk. Phos.	Mag.
Cal.	

PANCREATIC DYSFUNCTION, DEVELOPING

INCREASE	DECREASE
SGOT	Trig.
LDH	Cal.

PARASITES

INCREASE	DECREASE
EOS	Serum Iron
Occult Blood (Stool)	MCH
Total Glob.	MCHC
IgE	MCV
	HGB
	HCT
	RBC

PHLEBITIS

INCREASE	DECREASE
ALP	Lymphs
WBC	
SGOT	
EOS	
Neut.	
Acid Phos.	

POLYCYTHEMIA

INCREASE	DECREASE
HGB	MCH
HCT	MCV
Bili.	MCHC
Platlets	Iron
EOS	
WBC	
Uric Acid	

POSTERIOR PITUITARY DYSFUNCTION

INCREASE	DECREASE
Alt. BUN/Creat. Ratio	
Urinary Analysis (Specific gravity pH, osmolality)	

PROSTATE HYPERTROPHY, BENIGN

INCREASE	DECREASE
Creat.	
Acid Phos.	
Mono.	
Progosterone	
BUN	
Uric Acid	
Testosterone	

PROTEIN MALNUTRITION

INCREASE	DECREASE
B-12	Total Protein
	BUN
	HCT/HGB
	Alb.
	WBC
	Iron
	Cal.
	Mag.
	Potassium
	Alk. Phos.
	Beta/Gamma Glob.
	A/G Ratio

PYLORIC SPASM

INCREASE	DECREASE
Gastrin	Chlor.
	Potassium
	Sodium

RENAL DYSFUNCTION

INCREASE	DECREASE
Creat.	CO2
Acid Phos.	Cal.
Chlor.	Alb.
Phos.	HCT/HGB
BUN	
Uric Acid	
LDH	
SGOT	

RESPIRATORY DISTRESS

INCREASE	DECREASE
Alt. Chlor.	Bili.
Total Protein	Cort.
BUN	
Uric Acid	
Potassium	
Trig.	

RHEUMATOID ARTHRITIS

INCREASE	DECREASE
Alk. Phos.	SGOT
ESR	Alb.
Gamma Glob.	HCT/HGB
Neut.	
Platlets	
BUN	
Uric Acid	

RUBELLA

INCREASE	DECREASE
Lymphs	Platlets
	Neut.
	WBC

SHINGLES

INCREASE	DECREASE
ALP	Alb.
BUN	Chol.
LDH	
Mono.	
Creat.	

THYMUS DYSFUNCTION (HYPO ACTIVITY)

INCREASE	DECREASE
Bili.	
HGB	
HCT	
RBC	

WHOPPING COUGH (PERTUSSIS)

INCREASE	DECREASE
WBC	Neut.
Lymphs	

Systemic Formulas Catalog & Product Use Guide

SYSTEMIC FORMULAS SECTION

SYSTEMIC PRODUCT GUIDE

BIO COMMAND FORMULAS, Yellow Labels

#1	**Activator**	Use with a Bio Function formula to stimulate and activate the target organ or system. Note: Do not use in cases of infection or degeneration, but rather use #3, #4, or #5 first.
#2	**Builder**	Use with a Bio Function formula to strengthen, tonify, and rebuild the target organ or system.
#3	**Anti-Infective**	A general anti-infective and specific anti-bacterial formula. #3 Bolsters the body's natural defenses. It can be used by itself, or with a Bio Function. For deeper-seated conditions, #3 goes well with #435 GOLD or #403 ATAK.
#4	**Corrector**	A general anti-fungal and specific anti-candida, anti-yeast formula. Can be used by itself, or with a Bio Function.
#5	**Stabilizer**	Use with a Bio Function formula or with #483 OXCC to re-establish normal cellular health and integrity. Very effective in cases of cellular degeneration.
#6	**Healer**	Use with a Bio Function formula to stimulate healing and repair of damaged or weakened tissue.

BIO FUNCTION FORMULAS, Orange Labels

#12	**B**	**Brain**	A stimulant for superior mental functioning and to improve concentration, memory, and verbal skills. Ideal for students and for mental alertness.
#14	**C**	**Colon**	Rebuilds and tonifies intestinal function and peristaltic activity. It is both a gentle cleanser, and builder for many colon problems. Promotes regular elimination patterns.
#17	**D**	**Digestive**	A broad spectrum digestive aid when taken with meals. Taken between meals, it acts as a cleanser of the circulatory systems, both blood and lymphatic.
#18	**Ds**	**Digestive Stabilizer**	An unsurpassed digestive aid for the digestion of proteins, fats (oils), and carbohydrates. Soothing to the stomach.
#22	**F+**	**Female Plus**	The #1 formula for the ladies. F+ regulates and normalizes the female hormonal system and menstrual cycle. Effective for nine out of ten women.
#24	**Fpms**	**Female Premenses Syndrome**	For the more difficult PMS problems. Fpms is generally used with #22 F+.
#31	**Ga**	**Adrenal**	The pre-eminent energizer. A dynamic source of energy for the adrenals, and general body vitality. Also supports kidney function and assists in pH regulation, particularly when the pH is overly acid.
#32	**Gb**	**Pituitary**	Nutritional support for both the anterior and posterior pituitary as the "master gland." Goes well with #12 Brain and #50 Eyes.
#39	**Gf**	**Thyroid**	An effective and wonderful alternative to synthetic thyroid. Superb for hypo (low) thyroid. Also helps the body adjust to changes in climate and temperature.
#41	**Gt**	**Thymus**	The pre-eminent immune building formula. Strengthens the body's defenses and especially the thymus, spleen, liver, and lungs. Do <u>not</u> use for children under 12 years old, or for AIDS patients.
#44	**H**	**Heart**	A vigorous formula for strengthening the heart muscle and increasing stamina. Very powerful, use only one a day. Use <u>after</u> taking #45 Hcv first for two weeks.
#45	**Hcv**	**Cardiovascular**	Paramount nutritional support for circulatory health. Hcv normalizes blood pressure and helps remove arterial plaque and mineral deposition.

#46	Hn	Heart Nerve	Hn supports the bundle branch nerves to the heart as well as supporting and rebuilding the central nervous system as a whole. Used very successfully in cases of nerve damage, accidents, and trauma.
#50	I	Eyes	Supplies 28,000 IU vitamin A (fish source) per capsule, plus potent synergistic herbs to promote superior vision. Also strengthens the optical center of the brain (rear brain). Great for night driving.
#56	K	Kidney	Supports, strengthens, and rebuilds kidney function with a dynamic combination of vitamins, minerals, herbs, and free form amino acids.
#58	Ks	Kidney Stabilizer	Helps boost sluggish kidney and bladder function. Ks also assists maintain pH balance.
#60	L	Liver	The most comprehensive liver building formula available anywhere today. Nourishes, softens, and rebuilds the liver function. Far superior to milk thistle.
#61	Lb	Liver Normalizer	A specific for the gall bladder and portal duct to the liver. Lb builds the blood and helps in processing fats and oils. Very effective for hemorrhoids and varicosities.
#62	Ls	Liver Stimulant	The world's most dynamic liver detoxification and cleansing formula. Ls speeds up the natural healing process of the liver.
#70	M+	Male/Endocrine	A superior source of nutrition for the male glandular system. An energizer as well as a source of stamina and vitality. M+ also contains anti-inflammatory herbs to protect the prostate.
#72	Mpc	Prostata Corrector	A specific for candida or fungus of the prostate. Mpc helps relieve prostate congestion.
#73	Mpr	Prostata Ovatum	Lubricates, softens, and nourishes the prostate, ovaries and all the glands and joints of the body. A superior source of essential fatty acids from pumpkin seed oil.
#75	N-3	Anti-Tensive	Herbal, nutritional support for relief of nerve pain. Also used to help promote a more restful sleep.
#77	Nc	Calm	Soothes and calms the nerves, without harmful side effects. Nc is a superior, natural anti-stress formula.
#78	P	Pancreas	A pancreas builder which helps reduce blood glucose levels and control hyperglycemia.
#79	Ps	Pancreas Stabilizer	A superb formula for hypoglycemia. Ps boosts blood sugar levels smoothly and promptly.

#80	**R**	**Lung**	Nutritional support for the entire respiratory system, throat, bronchials, and lungs. Highly effective for asthma, smoker's cough, pneumonia, etc.
#81	**S**	**Spleen**	The first truly effective spleen formula in the Western world. Helps boost immune function, and the spleen's ability to filter the lymphatic and blood fluids.

BIO NUTRIMENT FORMULAS, Blue Label

#101	**ACP**	**Vitamin ACP**	A source of vitamins A, C, E, and P (Bioflavonoids) with specific herbs to strengthen the body's connective tissue (collagen). ACP also helps build resistance and accelerate the healing process.
#102	**ACX**	**Detoxifier**	A potent toxin neutralizer. Recommended with <u>any</u> cleansing program. ACX helps detoxify the body without adverse reactions or side effects.
#111	**AZV**	**Multi Vitamin**	AZV is the finest single multi-vitamin supplement available today. Patients really feel the difference when they take this superb formula.
#115	**BSV**	**Vitamin B Stress Complex**	A robust, high potency, yeast free, hypo-allergenic B-complex with vitalizing herbs. Provides ready energy.
#120	**CAL**	**Calcium Plus**	The most easily assimilated calcium supplement. Provides 9 different high quality calcium sources with magnesium, betaine Hcl, lecithin, vitamins D and E, iron, and boron.
#126	**CTV**	**Vitamin C Therapeutic**	A naturally buffered vitamin C complex along with anti-infective and detoxifying factors. Contains 450 mg. vitamin C, but is equivalent to 700 mg. in effect.
#130	**EZV**	**Vitamin E**	Totally natural, vitamin E from seed germ. EZV is in chewable form for sublingual assimilation to avoid destruction by stomach acids.
#134	**LEV**	**Lecithin 1200 mg.**	Rich in inositol, choline, and phospholipids for the health of every cell, especially the brain, heart, liver, and nerves.
#140	**MIN**	**Multi Mineral Plus**	The first herbal chelation mineral formula ever created. Supplies all trace minerals plus electrolytes. Superb for the heart, nerves, and glands.
#150	**PRO**	**Nutro-Protein**	Supplies the amino acids most often deficient in our diet today. PRO also helps the body utilize protein better.

BIO EXTRACT FORMULAS, Liquids

#200	AO	Aloe Vera	A highly concentrated aloe from the inner leaf of the famous aloe vera plant. AO possesses potent healing qualities. For internal as well as external use. AO promotes gastro-intestinal and skin health.
#225	EE	Escene Essence Oil	An analgesic, this soothing and healing oil brings prompt relief for aches, pain, and bruises.
#241	EV	Elixer Vita	A liquid tonic containing goldenseal, echinacea, and other herbs to strengthen the body's natural defenses as well as general vitality.
#250	TR	Tai Ra Chi	A dynamic, energetic extract which strengthens the body on a cellular level, and increases the electrical conductivity of the body. Also a specific for candida and fungus.
#260	WO	China Healing Oil	This Wonder Oil is often called "the first aid kit in a bottle". WO possesses powerful anti-infective and anti-inflammatory qualities, and accelerates healing. WO works overnight for sore throats, ear infections, burns, wounds, food poisoning, and 101 other uses.
#270	XL	Cleanser	An effective skin cleanser for acne and skin eruptions. XL is also very popular with the ladies as a most effective douche for yeast infections.

BIO PATHIC FORMULAS, Homeopathic Liquids

#325	COLD	Cold Stop	Contains homeopathic factors with zinc and methionine in an aqueous base. Helps prevent or alleviate cold and flu symptoms. Very effective at the onset of a cold.
#330	CTRC	Eyedrops	Effective in soothing tired, overworked eyes and for contact lens wearers. Has anti-flammatory, anti-infective qualities. Also effective in cataract prevention.

BIO CHALLENGE FORMULAS, Magenta Labels

#400	**APHA pH Control**	A pH buffer and adjustor especially for alkalosis (overly alkaline condition). A mild stimulant to the bowel and reduces excess mucous. Works well with #14 C-Colon.
#402	**ARTA Arthro Support**	The primary formula for arthritis and joint disorders. Relieves pain, stiffness, and affords welcome relief. Contains natural pain relievers, calcium metabolizers, and improves circulation.
#403	**ATAK Defense Rejuvenator**	Stimulates the body's natural defense systems. Formula ATAK unlocks subclinical pockets of infection, allowing the body's defenses to eliminate them. ATAK is generally used with an anti-infective formula such as GOLD, VIVI, #3, or #4 to eliminate the infection.
#405	**BLDB Blood Builder**	Supplies the herbal factors necessary to tonify and build strong blood. Helps improve the general quality of the blood.
#408	**CLNZ Toxin Chelator**	Unsurpassed in its ability to remove toxic heavy metals such as aluminum, mercury, lead, nickel, etc. as well as a variety of chemicals and poisons. Use with #126 CTV and #130 EZV.
#420	**DCSU Digestant Corrector**	Extremely effective for ulcers, shingles, and stomach pain, including hyperacidity. Calms and relaxes an upset stomach. DCSU also promotes rapid repair of damaged tissue anywhere in the body. For the elderly or if abnormal cell conditions are present, use #428 DSIR instead.
#425	**DIJS Stomach Antacid**	Quick relief for a sensitive stomach, acid indigestion, or acid rebound (heartburn). Helps reprogram the digestive system to establish the proper environment for good digestion. Helps break the commercial antacid habit.
#428	**DSIR Digestant-Internal Regenerator**	Activates the body's natural healing mechanisms by providing the building blocks for cell restructuring and to rebuild cell membranes. Accelerates recuperation following any surgery, accident, or trauma. Effective for the GI tract, as well as the whole body.
#435	**GOLD Defense Plus**	Many doctors call GOLD "the herbal antibiotic." It is a powerful antibacterial for infection, staph, strep, fever, etc. GOLD does <u>not</u> destroy the friendly bacterial flora, only pathogenic bacteria.
#450	**KDIR Diuretic**	A specific for breaking up and removing calcification and accumulation of mineral salts, gravel, and stones in the kidneys. Also assists in water retention. Generally used <u>with</u> formula K.

#460	**KYRO Muscle/Ligament Strength**	Supplies bountiful nutritional factors to strengthen the soft tissue of the body. Assists the patient to hold chiropractic adjustments longer and better.
#481	**OXAA Cell Organizer**	Similar to #483 OXOX, but with additional support for the liver. OXAA is especially important for oxygenating the deep tissues such as lungs, breast, and bone.
#482	**OXCC Cell Cleanser**	A deep cleansing and detoxification formula with oxygenating and cell normalizing qualities. Helps eliminate degenerative and abnormal cells. Works well with #5 stabilizer.
#483	**OXOX Cell Activator**	A cellular oxygenator which encourages elimination of cellular toxins. OXOX is good as a general cleanser as well as for general malaise.
#486	**SENG Red Ginseng +**	A stimulant for both the glandular and lymphatic systems. SENG cleans and stimulates the lymphatics. It is especially good at removing lymphatic congestion.
#488	**VIVI Anti-Viro**	Stong anti-viral action. Effective for flu, colds, herpes, and most viral strains. Even more effective with #403 ATAK, for the more chronic viral problems.
#490	**VRM1 Para-Large**	Powerful vermifuge for the larger variety of parasites (such as tapeworms) which infect the large intestine.
#491	**VRM2 Para-Small**	For smaller parasites (such as roundworms), and parasites that are beyond the intestinal tract. Also effective for pets.
#492	**VRM3 Para-Micro**	For waterborne and microscopic parasites such as giardiasis (Giardia lamblia), or amoebas (Entamoeba Histolytica). Use with 3-6 drops #260 WO, in an empty capsule.
#493	**VRM4 Para-Cell**	For kidney or liver flukes or blastocystis hominis. Also effective for amoebas in certain cases. Use with 3-6 drops #260 WO, in an empty capsule.

PRODUCT DIRECTIONS FOR HEALTH PROFESSIONALS

The following information provides general guidelines to doctors. Actual dosages may vary from day to day, and are best determined with each patient.

In general, the **Systemic Formulas** work best when taken away from food, between meals. However, all the formulas (except for L, Ls and S) can be used at anytime, if needed or required. Formulas L, Ls and S must always be taken away from food to derive benefit, at least 1 hour before or 2 hours after eating.

Fine\Delicate mannerism individuals (more sensitive types with thinner skin, smaller bone structure and finer hair) generally require smaller dosages. **Coarse\Robust mannerism individuals** (stronger body types with thicker skin, larger bone structure, and coarser hair) may take slightly larger dosages.

Systemic Formulas are "self-limiting." They support and rebuild organ and body systems without requiring an endless supply of that same formula, month after month. The Master Matrix of each formula provides cellular identity factors (RNA-DNA) to re-establish a dynamic equilibrium (homeostasis) within the body. This generally occurs within 1-3 months of using a formula. After homeostasis is achieved the formula may be discontinued, or used on an occasional basis, as needed. Of course, general maintenance formulas such as AZV (Multi Vitamin), MIN (Multi Mineral), and BSV (Vitamin B Stress Complex) may be used daily.

NOTES

(†) Formula #4 (Corrector) may produce a cleansing reaction, if the patient proceeds too quickly in its use. It is better to start slowly and gradually increase dosage. ACP or ACX may be helpful also, to neutralize toxins being eliminated.

(††) Formulas ACP and ACX are recommended in any cleansing program. They help neutralize toxins and wastes, and minimize any healing crisis or reaction, especially with the sensitive-type patient. They are recommended with programs that use Formulas #4 (Corrector), ATAK, OXOX, OXAA, OXCC, or any the of the VRM formulas. Generally ACP is used with the young, weak, or elderly. ACX is used in most other cases.

(†††) Kidney or liver functions may require strengthening (with Formulas K or L) before or while using one of the VRM formulas. As with any cleansing program, the elimination system must be kept open. Drink at least 1 quart water daily. Formulas ACP or ACX are used to aid the cleansing process as a toxin neutralizer. Also 1 bottle of DCSU or DSIR is recommended after completing the VRM program, to aid in tissue healing.

Do not begin a VRM program unless the patient plans to complete it entirely. Do not use any VRM formula if abdominal pain, cramps, nausea, or other signs of appendicitis are present. Do not use during pregnancy, while nursing, or for children under the age of six (age eight for the use of the VRM1 formula). Do not eat beef or pork while on this program. Fish or poultry may be eaten in moderation.

SPECIAL NOTE

When using any of the anti-infective formulas (#3, #4, GOLD, ATAK, VIVI), it is best to continue their use for 10-14 days after all symptoms and signs of infection are gone. This strengthens the body and helps assure that the infection does not return.

BIO COMMAND FORMULAS

PRODUCT			W/ FOOD		RECOMMENDED USAGE		AVG. LENGTH OF PROGRAM	ADDITIONAL NOTES
No.	CODE	NAME	YES	NO	Fine/Delicate Mannerism	Coarse/Robust Mannerism		
#1	1	ACTIVATOR		•	1 capsule with a BioFunction Formula, 1-2 times daily.	1-2 capsules w/ a BioFunction Formula, 1-2 times daily.	2 to 4 weeks.	Caution: Use Formulas #3 and #4 first if signs of infection, virus or degeneration are present.
#2	2	BUILDER		•	1 capsule with a BioFunction Formula, 1-2 times daily.	1-2 capsules with BioFunction Formula, 1-2 times daily.	2 to 4 weeks.	May be used with DCSU to promote deep tissue rebuilding.
#3	3	ANTI-INFECTIVE		•	1-2 capsules alone or with a BioFunction Formula, 1-3 times a day.	2-3 capsules alone or with a BioFunction Formula, 1-4 times a day.	2 to 4 weeks.	May be alternated with GOLD every other week. Use with GOLD and/or ATAK for deeper type infections.
#4	4	CORRECTOR (†)		•	1 capsule alone or with a BioFunction Formula, 1-3 times a day	1-2 capsule alone or with a BioFunction Formula, 1-3 times a day.	1-3 months and then as needed for maintenance.	Start w/ 1 capsule daily and slowly increase dosage. Use w/ ATAK for chronic conditions.
#5	5	STABILIZER		•	1 capsule with a BioFunction Formula, 1-2 times a day.	2-3 capsules with a BioFunction Formula, 1-3 times a day.	2 to 4 weeks.	May be used with Formulas OXOX, OXAA, OXCC
#6	6	HEALER		•	1 capsule with a BioFunction Formula, 1-2 times a day.	2 capsules with a BioFunction Formula, 1-3 times a day.	2 to 4 weeks.	Healing accelerant. May be used w/DCSU to assist in ulcerative conditions of stomach/intestine

BIO FUNCTION FORMULAS

PRODUCT			W/ FOOD		RECOMMENDED USAGE		AVG. LENGTH OF PROGRAM	ADDITIONAL NOTES
No.	CODE	NAME	YES	NO	Fine/Delicate Mannerism	Coarse/Robust Mannerism		
#12	B	BRAIN		•	1-2 capsules once a day.	2 capsules, 1-2 times a day.	1-3 months and then as needed for maintenance.	Works well w/ Formulas I, Gb. Excellent for hyperactive children, mental clarity, etc.
#14	C	COLON	•	•	1-2 capsules, 1-2 times a day.	1-2 capsules, 1-2 times a day.	1-6 months and then as needed for maintenance.	A mild colon cleansing formula; strengthens peristaltic action and builds colon function.
#17	D	DIGESTIVE	•	•	1 capsule, 1-2 times a day.	1-2 capsules, 1-2 times a day.	1-3 months and then as needed for maintenance.	To assist digestion take with meals; to lower cholesterol take 1 capsule between meals, with liquids.
#18	Ds	DIGEST STABILIZER	•		1 tablet; 1-2 times a day.	1-2 tablets, 1-2 times a day.	1-3 months and then as needed for maintenance.	Milder form of Formula D; excellent digestant.

PRODUCT			W/ FOOD		RECOMMENDED USAGE		AVG. LENGTH OF PROGRAM	ADDITIONAL NOTES
No.	CODE	NAME	YES	NO	Fine/Delicate Mannerism	Coarse/Robust Mannerism		
#22	F+	FEMALE PLUS		•	1-2 capsules; 1-2 times a day (best upon arising).	2 capsules; 1-2 times a day (best upon arising).	1-4 months and then as needed for maintenance.	May be used with Gb, Mpr or Fpms; regulates female bio-chemistry.
#24	Fpms	FEMALE PREMENSES SYNDROME		•	1-2 capsules; 1-2 times a day.	2 capsules; 1-2 times a day.	1-4 months and then as needed for maintenance.	Works well with F+; helps to normalize menstrual cycle and decrease symptoms without side effects.
#31	Ga	ADRENAL	•	•	1 capsule; 1-2 times a day; best when taken mid-morning and mid-afternoon.	2 capsules; 1-2 times a day best when taken mid-morning and mid-afternoon.	1-3 months and then as needed for maintenance.	Works well with Gb, Gf, Gt, K or Ks; to stop an acid pH cycle take 1 Ga with 2 N2, at bedtime.
#32	Gb	PITUITARY		•	1 capsule; 1-2 times a day.	1-2 capsules; 1-2 times a day.	1-3 months and then as needed for maintenance.	It complements B, I, Ga, Gf, Gt, F+ and M+; also supports pineal and thalamus.
#39	Gf	THYROID	•	•	1 capsule; 1-2 times a day.	1-2 capsules; 1-2 times a day.	1-4 months and then as needed for maintenance.	Works well with Ga, Gb, Gt, and F+; for jet-leg take 3 capsules before flight and 3 upon landing.
#41	Gt	THYMUS		•	1 capsule; 1-2 times a day.	1-2 capsules; 1-3 times a day.	1-3 months and then as needed for maintenance.	A superior Formula for strengthening the body's immune system.
#44	H	HEART	•	•	1 capsule; once a day.	1 capsule; 1-2 times a day.	1-3 months and then as needed for maintenance.	Builds body stamina; strengthens healthy heart; use Hcv for two weeks <u>prior</u> to Formula H .
#45	Hcv	CARDIO VASCULAR		•	1-2 capsules; 1-2 times a day.	2 capsules; 1-2 times a day.	1-3 months and then as needed for maintenance.	It helps to strengthen blood vessels and remove arterial plaques.
#46	Hn	HEART NERVE	•	•	1 capsule; 1-2 times a day.	2-3 capsules; 1-2 times a day.	1-9 months and then as needed for maintenance.	Repairs and restores the bundle branch nerves to the heart and the nerve system in general.
#50	I	EYES	•	•	1-2 capsules; 1-2 times a day.	1-3 capsules; 1-2 times a day.	1-4 months and then as needed for maintenance.	Works well with Formulas B and Gb; also with #4 and ATAK to prevent colds; supports optic center of the brain.
#56	K	KIDNEY (†††)	•	•	1-2 capsules; 1-2 times a day.	2 capsules; 1-2 times a day.	1-4 months and then as needed for maintenance.	Profound kidney support; often relieves lower back pain; works well with DSIR or ACX.

PRODUCT			W/ FOOD		RECOMMENDED USAGE		AVG. LENGTH OF PROGRAM	ADDITIONAL NOTES
No.	CODE	NAME	YES	NO	Fine/Delicate Mannerism	Coarse/Robust Mannerism		
#58	Ks	KIDNEY STABILIZER	•	•	1-2 tablets; 1-2 times a day.	2-4 tablets; 1-2 times a day.	1-3 months and then as needed for maintenance.	Milder form of Formula K for long term kidney support; alternate with K.
#60	L	LIVER (†††)		•	1-2 capsules; 1-2 times a day.	2 capsules; 1-2 times a day.	1-6 months and then as needed for maintenance.	Total support for the liver and gall bladder; must be taken at least 2 hs after or 1 hr before eating; goes well with Lb, Ls, S.
#61	Lb	LIVER NORMALIZER		•	1-2 tablets; 1-2 times a day.	2-3 tablets; 1-2 times a day.	1-3 months and then as needed for maintenance.	Goes well with L, Ls; for hemorrhoids also eat 1 small raw red beet daily.
#62	Ls	LIVER STIMULANT		•	1 capsule; once a day.	1-2 capsules; 1-2 times a day.	1-3 months and then as needed for maintenance.	Must be taken at least 2 hs after or 1 hr before food; goes well with L and S.
#70	M+	SUPERMALE		•	1-2 capsules; 1-2 times daily.	2 capsules; 1-2 times daily.	1-6 months and then as needed for maintenance.	For the male endocrine system; also to increase overall circulation; good with Mpr.
#72	Mpc	PROSTATA CORRECTOR		•	1-2 hard capsules; 1-2 times a day. Ratio: 1 soft pill for each 3 hard capsules.	2 hard capsules; 1-2 times a day. Ratio: 1 soft pill for each 3 hard capsules.	1-6 months and then as needed for maintenance.	For men to counteract candida of prostate. Goes well with TR.
#73	Mpr	PROSTATA/ /OVATUM	•	•	1 capsule; 1-2 times a day.	1-2 capsules; 1-2 times a day.	1-6 months and then as needed for maintenance.	Works well with M+, Mpc, F+ and Gb.
#76	N2	ANTI-NEURO		•	1-2 capsules; 1-2 times a day.	2 capsules; 1-2 times a day.	1-3 months and then as needed for maintenance.	To aid sleep take 1-2 capsules 1 hr before bed. Works well w/Ga for chronic acidosis (urine pH).
#77	Nc	CALM		•	1-2 capsules; 1-3 times a day.	2 capsules; 1-3 times a day.	1-3 months and then as needed .	Calms the nerves; to quiet stomach take 1-2 capsules 20 min before eating.
#78	P	PANCREAS	•	•	1-2 capsules; 1-2 times a day.	2 capsules; 1-2 times a day.	1-4 months and then as needed for maintenance.	Best if taken PM, between meals.
#79	Ps	PANCREAS STABILIZER	•	•	1-2 capsules; 1-2 times a day.	2 capsules; 1-2 times a day.	1-4 months and then as needed for maintenance.	Best early in the day between meals; regulates blood sugar. levels.

PRODUCT			W/ FOOD		RECOMMENDED USAGE		AVG. LENGTH OF PROGRAM	ADDITIONAL NOTES
No.	CODE	NAME	YES	NO	Fine/Delicate Mannerism	Coarse/Robust Mannerism		
#80	R	LUNG		•	1-2 capsules; 1-2 times a day.	2 capsules; 1-2 times a day.	1-3 months and then as needed for maintenance.	Works well w/ #3, #4, ATAK, VIVI; complementary Formulas are C and APHA.
#82	S	SPLEEN		•	1-2 capsules; 1-2 times a day.	2 capsules; 1-2 times a day.	1-3 months and then as needed for maintenance.	Must be taken at least 2 hrs after or 1 hr before food; goes well with L, Ls and ACX.

BIO NUTRIMENT FORMULAS

PRODUCT			W/ FOOD		RECOMMENDED USAGE		AVG. LENGTH OF PROGRAM	ADDITIONAL NOTES
No.	CODE	NAME	YES	NO	Fine/Delicate Mannerism	Coarse/Robust Mannerism		
#101	ACP	VITAMIN ACP (†)(††)(†††)	•	•	1-2 capsules; 1-3 times a day.	2-3 capsules; 1-3 times a day.	1-3 months and then as needed .	Builds collagen and tissue integrity; strengthens immunity; good on any cleansing program.
#102	ACX	VITAMIN DETOX (†)(††)(†††)	•	•	1-2 capsules; 1-3 times a day.	2 capsules; 1-3 times a day.	1-2 months and then as needed for maintenance.	Excellent all purpose detoxifier; helps to neutralize cleansing reaction of any kind.
#111	AZV	MULTI-VITAMIN	•		1 light + 1 dark capsule a day.	1 light + 1 dark capsule a day.	Daily as general maintenance.	The one multi-vitamin/mineral in which people really feel the difference. It energizes.
#115	BSV	VITAMIN B STRESS COMPLEX	•	•	1 capsule; 1-2 times a day.	1-2 capsules; 1-2 times a day.	Daily as general maintenance.	A robust allergin-free, yeast-free B-Complex with vitalizing herbs for maximum assimilation.
#120	CAL	CALCIUM-PLUS	•	•	1 tablet; 1-2 times a day. (Best <u>before</u> breakfast)	1-2 tablets; 1-3 times a day. (Best <u>before</u> breakfast)	Daily as general maintenance.	Nine different sources of Calcium with Magnesium and Vitamins C, D and E, plus Lecithin.
#126	CTV	VITAMIN C THERAPEUTIC	•	•	1-2 caplets; 1-4 times a day.	1-2 caplets; 1-4 times a day.	Daily as general maintenance.	Five different sources of Vit. C with Vit. A and Calcium, Potassium, Thymol Iodide.
#130	EZV	200 IU VIT. E	•	•	Chew 1-2 tablets; 1-3 times a day.	Chew 1-2 tablets; 1-3 times a day.	Daily as general maintenance.	Truly 100% natural Vit. E; Its chewable form optimizes assimilation; best between meals.
#134	LEV	LECITHIN	•	•	1-2 capsules; 1-2 times a day.	1-2 capsules; 1-2 times a day.	Daily as general maintenance.	Goes well with N2 or Nc for a restful sleep; for higher doses use with CAL.
#140	MIN	MULTI-MINERAL	•	•	1 capsule; 1-2 times a day.	1-2 capsules; 1-2 times a day.	Daily as general maintenance.	The only herbal chelation mineral formula available today; best in early part of the day.

PRODUCT			W/ FOOD		RECOMMENDED USAGE		AVG. LENGTH OF PROGRAM	ADDITIONAL NOTES
No.	CODE	NAME	YES	NO	Fine/Delicate Mannerism	Coarse/Robust Mannerism		
#150	PRO	NUTRO PROTEIN	•	•	1-2 capsules; 1-2 times a day.	1-2 capsules; 1-2 times a day.	Daily as general maintenance.	Provides essential amino-acids commonly deficient in today's diet; enhances and completes the protein structure.

BIO EXTRACT FORMULAS

PRODUCT			W/ FOOD		RECOMMENDED USAGE		AVG. LENGTH OF PROGRAM	ADDITIONAL NOTES
No.	CODE	NAME	YES	NO	Fine/Delicate Mannerism	Coarse/Robust Mannerism		
#200	AO	ALOE VERA		•	Internally: 1-3 Tbsp in water; 1-2 times a day. Externally: Apply full strength.	Internally: 1-3 Tbsp in water; 1-2 times a day Externally: Apply full strength.	1-4 months and then as needed for maintenance.	A 4 times concentrate of the inner leaves of the Aloe Vera plant; potent healing qualities.
#225	EE	ESSENE OIL	•	•	Topically, or 1-4 drops in a glass of water.	Topically, or 1-4 drops in a glass of water.	1-8 weeks or as needed.	Helps set adjustments. Caution: Keep out of mucous membrane.
#240	EV	ELIXER VITA	•	•	3-5 drops, 1-3 times a day, orally, or in a glass of water.	6-15 drops, 2-4 times a day, orally or in a glass of water.	4 weeks or as needed.	Fights bacterial infections and helps cleanse the system.
#250	TR	TAI RA CHI	•	•	1-3 drops under tongue; 1-3 times a day.	2-30 drops under tongue; 1-3 times a day.	1-4 months and then as needed for maintenance.	Start with only 1-2 drops at a time and gradually increase; may be added to water or juice.
#260	WO	HEALING OIL	•	•	Topically, or 1-4 drops in a glass of water.	Topically, or 1-6 drops in a glass of water.	1-4 weeks or as needed.	A first aid station in a bottle; Anti-infective. Caution: Keep out of mucous membranes.
#270	XL	CLEANSER	•	•	Use externally only. Dilute 1 part XL to 10 parts of water.	Use externally only. Dilute 1 part XL to 10 parts of water.	1-2 weeks and then as needed.	For acne, skin rashes, poisoning Ivy and Oak, etc. For douche: 1 Tbsp of XL w/ 1 pint of water.

BIO PATHIC FORMULAS

PRODUCT			W/ FOOD		RECOMMENDED USAGE		AVG. LENGTH OF PROGRAM	ADDITIONAL NOTES
No.	CODE	NAME	YES	NO	Fine/Delicate Mannerism	Coarse/Robust Mannerism		
#325	COLD	COLD STOP	•	•	1-4 drops; 3-4 times a day.	1-6 drops; 3-4 times a day.	Occasional use as needed.	Aids in the prevention/relief of cold symptoms and sore throats.
#330	CTRC	CATARACT	•	•	1-2 drops in each eye; 1-4 times a day.	1-2 drops in each eye; 1-4 times a day.	1-4 months and then as needed for maintenance.	Many who wear contact lenses find CTRC very soothing; helps clear eye irritation.

BIO CHALLENGE FORMULAS

PRODUCT			W/ FOOD		RECOMMENDED USAGE		AVG. LENGTH OF PROGRAM	ADDITIONAL NOTES
No.	CODE	NAME	YES	NO	Fine/Delicate Mannerism	Coarse/Robust Mannerism		
#400	APHA	pH CONTROL		•	1-2 capsules; 1-2 times a day.	2 capsules; 1-2 times a day.	Occasional use as needed to balance pH.	Works well with Formula C; neutralizes alkalosis.
#402	ARTA	ARTHRO SUPPORT	•	•	1-2 capsules; 1-2 times a day. (Best with food)	2-4 capsules; 1-2 times a day. (Best with food)	1-4 months and then as needed for maintenance.	Very compatible with N2 when joint pain is present. Use also EE topically.
#403	ATAK	DEFENSE REJUVENATOR (††)		•	1 capsule; 1-2 times a day.	1-2 capsules; 1-2 times a day.	1-3 months and then as needed for maintenance.	Generally used with GOLD or #4; ATAK breaks loose pockets of cellular toxins and GOLD or #4 neutralizes and eliminates them.
#405	BLDB	BLOOD BUILDER		•	1-2 capsules; 1-2 times a day.	2 capsules; 1-2 times a day.	1-2 months and then as needed for maintenance.	Supplies nutrients and organic iron to blood stream.
#408	CLNZ	TOXIN CHELATOR		•	1 capsule; 1-2 times a day.	2 capsules; 1-2 times a day.	1-2 months and then as needed for maintenance.	Purifies and detoxifies the blood while chelating out heavy metals.
#420	DCSU	DIGESTA-SOOTHER (†††)		•	2 tablets up to 15 times a day.	2 tablets up to 15 times a day.	1-3 weeks and then as needed for maintenance.	Accelerates healing anywhere in the body; promotes prompt tissue repair.
#425	DIJS	STOMACH ANTACID		•	1-2 capsules; 1-3 times a day.	2 capsules; 1-3 times a day.	1-3 weeks and then as needed for maintenance.	Fifteen minutes before eating is best to help control acid in digestion, flatulence, etc.
#428	DSIR	DIGESTIVE-INTERNAL REGENERATOR		•	1-2 tablets; 1-2 times a day.	2 tablets; 1-3 times a day.	2-8 weeks and then as needed for maintenance.	Similar to DCSU, but does not contain Comfrey, thus use DSIR with abnormal cell situations.
#435	GOLD	DEFENSE PLUS	•	•	1 capsule only, 1-4 times a day.	1 capsule, 1-6 times a day. May increase to 2 capsules after 3-5 days. Caution: Niacin flush may occur.	2-4 weeks and then as needed for maintenance.	Take w/ food to minimize niacin flush; diabetics: use for 3 days only or use #3; Increase Vit. B intake with 1-2 BSV a day.
#450	KDIR	DIURETIC		•	1-2 capsules, 1-2 times a day.	2 capsules, 1-2 times a day.	2-8 weeks and then as needed for maintenance.	Works well with K or Ks for edema and pre-menstrual weight gain.
#460	KYRO	MUSCLE-LIGAMENT-TISSUE STRENGTHENER	•	•	1-2 capsules, once a day. (Best with food)	2-3 capsules, once a day. (Best with food)	1-6 months and then as needed for maintenance.	Support chiropractic adjustments so they will hold better and longer.

PRODUCT			W/ FOOD		RECOMMENDED USAGE		AVG. LENGTH OF PROGRAM	ADDITIONAL NOTES
No.	CODE	NAME	YES	NO	Fine/Delicate Mannerism	Coarse/Robust Mannerism		
#481	OXAA	CELL ORGANIZER (††)		•	1-2 capsules, 1-2 times a day.	2 capsules, 1-2 times a day.	1-4 months and then as needed for maintenance.	Upon arising or at bedtime; best away from food; compatible with #3, #4, #5, ATAK, OXOX and/ or specific BioFunction.
#482	OXCC	CELL NORMALIZER (††)		•	1-2 capsules, 1-2 times a day.	2 capsules, 1-2 times a day.	1-4 months and then as needed for maintenance.	Upon arising or at bedtime; best away from food; goes well with #3, #4, #5, ATAK, OXOX and/ or specific BioFunction.
#483	OXOX	CELL ACTIVATOR (††)		•	1-2 capsules, 1-2 times a day.	2 capsules, 1-2 times a day.	1-4 months and then as needed for maintenance.	May be used with #3, #4 or #5 and /or a specific BioFunction. Also compatible with OXAA, OXCC, ATAK for cell cleansing.
#486	SENG	RED GINSENG PLUS		•	1-2 capsules, 1-2 times a day.	2 capsules, 1-2 times a day.	1-2 months and then as needed for maintenance.	Highly effective lymphatic cleanser, gland toner and de-congestant.
#488	VIVI	ANTI-VIRO		•	1 capsule, 1-4 times a day.	2-3 capsules, 1-4 times a day.	2-4 weeks and then as needed for maintenance.	Fights any viral infection. Do not use if pregnant! Skin rash may rarely occur; if so correct pH (take a bath w/ 2 cups baking soda) & stop VIVI for 3 days.
#490	VRM1	PARA-LARGE (††)(†††)		•	1-2 capsules at bedtime.	2-3 capsules at bedtime.	4-6 cycles of 15 days each. **(see bottle)**	Sixty consecutive days is the minimum program (4 cycles of 15 days); but 90 days (6 cycles) may be required. May cause loose stool.
#491	VRM2	PARA-SMALL (††)(†††)		•	1-2 capsules at bedtime.	2-3 capsules at bedtime.	4-6 cycles of 15 days each. **(see bottle)**	Sixty consecutive days is the minimum program (4 cycles of 15 days); but 90 days (6 cycles) may be required. May cause loose stool.
#492	VRM3	PARA-MICRO (††)(†††)		•	1-2 capsules at bedtime.	2 capsules at bedtime. (3 capsules may be needed in specific cases)	30-75 days	Generally used with 3 drops of WO in a capsule. May cause loose stool.
#493	VRM4	PARA-CELL (††)(†††)		•	1-2 capsules at bedtime.	2 capsules at bedtime. (3 capsules may be needed in specific cases)	30-75 days	Generally used with 3 drops of WO in a capsule. May cause loose stool.

APPLE-A-DAY PRESS CATALOG

Natural Healing At Your Fingertips

Welcome to Apple-A-Day Press — your resource for natural health information featuring the insights of Dr. Jack Tips. Here you'll find informative books and training programs. Since 1984, *Apple-A-Day Press* has published books and natural health courses that have helped hundreds of thousands of people improve their health. Here you will find information congruent with the "Natural Laws of Life and Healing from the *causative* perspective." Best wishes in your health endeavors!

Apple-A-Day Press

1500 Village West Drive, Suite 77, Austin, Texas 78733

Phone: 512.328.3996 Fax: 512.263.7787

Website: www.apple-a-daypress.com

Email: apple-a-day@austin.rr.com

Toll Free Order Line (orders only, 24-hours secure): 877.442.7753

Web Site: www.apple-a-daypress.com

Download excerpts of these books, get free articles.

POPULAR BOOKS

The Weight Is Over by Dr. Jack Tips

A powerful, health-building book. The last weight-loss book you'll ever need to read. Much more than how to lose weight, this book teaches how to gain true health!

Anyone can benefit from this myth-busting breakthrough! Get trim now! It's not your fault your weight is up and your energy is down. You've avoided fat, you've increased grains, you've eaten less—just like they told you. But you know what? They told you wrong! Now, for the first time, find out why people have excessive weight and how you can eradicate it. Learn about the perfect, custom-designed eating plan for you as an individual! *The Weight Is Over* is a groundbreaking new program that takes you step by step into a mastery of nutrition—both eating to lose fat and building optimal health simultaneously. Much more than a crash program, this book helps you build a healthy lifestyle that will benefit you for the rest of your life. Learn about:

- So called "bad" foods that are really good for you!
- Super foods that unleash your body's ability to burn fat while you sleep!
- Herbs and nutrients that help you burn fat for energy!
- 'Syndrome X' and how it silently kills people.
- The 12 Optimal Food Factors—never before published insights on everything your diet must provide to prevent disease and bring health!

300 pages. ISBN 0-929167-21-X $24.95

Passion Play by Dr. Jack Tips

If ever a book could change your life — increase your wealth, improve your relationships, and open your heart — this is it. Absolutely profound and insightful. Believe this — the Mirror Technique is a true shortcut to success in any endeavor. It starts where other self-help books leave off — beyond affirmations, beyond visualization, beyond anything you've ever tried!

Passion Play is the art of combining Sensualization® with the Native American Mirror Technique to harness your hidden power of manifestation. Use this technique to awaken your heart, encourage your actions, enliven your dreams, clarify your mission, achieve your goals and discover your true destiny. *Passion Play* is a new, powerful breakthrough in self-realization and human potential. Wealth, love, romance, success, charity, health, freedom, contentment, joy, excitement and spiritual adventures await you—within these pages, within your life. Never before has the step-by-step process to recreate yourself, create your future life, and follow your heart's desire become so clear, simple, and effective. Now you can discover your passion and begin your play. Passion Play will improve your life...forever.

290 pages, ISBN 0-929167-20-1 $24.95

The Pro-Vital Plan for Optimal Nutrition by Dr. Jack Tips

A nutrition classic and one of the most important natural health books of the 20th Century! Absolutely a must read for every natural health practitioner and anyone wanting to end the confusion about dietary health.

Here is a simple and comprehensive way to build your health, prevent disease, and increase longevity based on both biochemistry and bio-energy! An extraordinary overview of how to minimize dietary stress and maximize utilization of the highest quality food factors: protein, fat, carbohydrates, minerals, vitamins, enzymes, fiber, and nascent water, and bio-energy. A safe, non-radical nutritional foundation based on the 'ancient wisdom' and 'horse sense' that can change your life and bring the best of health. Daily nutrition plans and delicious recipes are included. Learn how to design the optimal nutrition meal and turn your eating experience into a healing experience! You will gain a greater understanding of nutrition and its role in health. A simple approach to more energy, weight loss, improved immunity, and better health!

376 pages, index. ISBN 0-929167-05-8 $24.95

Conquer Candida—Restore Your Immune System by Dr. Jack Tips

Not just another candida book but a natural health milestone. This book goes where others have never dared—a deeper understanding of health and its restoration.

Hailed by readers and natural health practitioners alike as the finest and most easy to understand book about the "canary in the mine shaft" regarding your health. Not just another candida book, here is an in-depth look at the silent, health-undermining pandemic that contributes to allergies, chronic fatigue, PMS, chronic infections, headaches, bloating, memory loss, and immune deficiencies. More importantly, this book explains what to do about these conditions by indicating true causes and offering unique insights based on hundreds of clinical case histories. "Many people blame all their health ailments on candida (yeast fungus), but this is not really the problem! Many people overlook the fact that candida is not only a symptom of impaired immunity, it also predisposes people to further poor health and low energy. You cannot quickly win the battle against candida by dietary adjustment, but you can with proper natural health therapy." Find out if candida is a factor in your health picture and what to do about it. This information goes beyond current treatments and offers an understanding of how to truly conquer candida and restore your most optimal health.

163 pages. ISBN 0-929167-00-7 $15.95

Breast Health—A Women's Health Discourse by Dr. Jack Tips

Are you simply waiting and hoping your next mammogram won't steal your life with the dreaded news? Find out what you can do now not only to protect your health but to and have overall female hormone balance. Find out why men need to read this material, too.

From the natural health perspective, there are clear reasons that breast cancer occurs and thus there are clear steps to take to prevent it! In this discourse, you will learn the reasons that the breast tissue is susceptible to disease and learn simple steps to avoid them. Beyond disease concerns, the breasts play an important role in overall female hormonal balance. Breast health is an important part of overcoming PMS, menstrual cramping, endometriosis, and menopausal symptoms. This discourse discusses the role of breast tissue in female endocrine balance and demonstrates how to maintain healthy breast tissue. Features the breast-test and breast massage technique to help prevent breast disease and maintain tissue integrity.

56 pages, illustrations, $9.95

BOOKS & TAPES

The Next Step to Greater Energy—A Unique Perspective on Bioenergy, Addictions and Transformation by Dr. Jack Tips

Are your "little addictions" a clear symptom of a metabolic imbalance? Breaking addictive behaviors is more effective with this information.

Explore the energy systems of the body with emphasis on both the glandular (thyroid and adrenals) and bio-electric energy systems. This book presents a new look at the connection between bio-energy and addictions. Discover energy impostors including substances, activities, and habits. Identify addictions and habits as symptoms of bio-energetic and biochemical imbalances. Discover the true cause of cravings and addictive patterns, and how to correct the underlying imbalances. How to stop smoking is thoroughly discussed. The focus of this practical information is how to obtain freedom and fuller spiritual expression. 210 pages, index. Out of print. Available as web download or a CD file for you to read or print out.

ISBN 0-929167-04-X $16.95

The Healing Triad: Your Liver—Your Lifeline! by Dr. Jack Tips

This book discusses the most important organ in your body—the liver—and how to support and improve its function and detoxification capacity. This information changes lives! Fascinating insights on how to detoxify your entire body by building your inherent liver function.

Featured at Anthony Robbins' Life Mastery University, here is the key to detoxification and restoration of proper liver function. This is a fascinating look at the liver—your most important organ—its bio-force and the Chinese healing system involving the triad of the liver-stomach-colon. Explains in easy steps how to detoxify your liver, gall bladder and entire body the natural way. Contains provocative insights into how herbs really work to help your body heal. Reveals natural liver treatments and cures. Shows you how to build the very foundation upon which your health rests! Doc Wheelwright discovered seven miraculous herbs that support the complex liver systems and created a remarkable breakthrough in liver support. A *must read* for people with concerns regarding Hepatitis C and anyone wanting to live life in the best of health.

150 pages, illustrations, photos, index, ISBN 0-929167-06-6 $15.95

FOR THE HEALTH PROFESSIONAL

New Dimensions In Herbal Healing Training Program

by Drs. Jack Tips and Tim Kuss

Master the Doc Wheelwright healing formulas and learn his programming secrets with this professional training course that becomes your desk reference book for one of the most advanced healing systems in the world.

Learn the secrets of one of the 20th century's greatest herbal healers—A.S. "Doc" Wheelwright—and the Systemic formulas. Join two of his protégés—Dr. Jack Tips and Dr. Timothy Kuss—as they discuss the healing philosophies and practices that have made them nationally renowned practitioners. In this program, they teach the techniques and insights of natural health coupled with in-depth training in the applications of the Wheelwright Legacy—the unsurpassed Systemic herbal/nutritional formulations. This certification program will soon become your strongest ally in the most important facet of your natural health practice—true healing results! Reveals Wheelwright's secrets about how and why he created his famous herbal healing combinations. You will quickly become proficient in comprehensive program design using Wheelwright's complete healing system. This program will make you a master of systemic herbology.

19 CD's in binder, 350-page Desk Reference,
150-page Study Guide [List $799] now $599.

New Dimensions In Herbal Healing (Book) by Dr. Jack Tips

Finally! A book that explains the pioneering, bio-energetic, herbal research of one of the 20th century's great healers—A.S. Doc Wheelwright. Learn about the Wheelwright Healing System and how herbs are the true medicine for the challenges of living in the 21st Century. Focuses on the Bio-Commands – a method on how to provide a healing directive to herbal programs. Features protocols for the Kidneys, Thyroid, Brain Building, Heart Building, A.D.H.D., Liver, Cleansing, Female Hormonal Issues, and Lungs.

110 pages, ISBN 0-929167-23-6 $19.95

Blood Chemistry & Clinical Nutrition by Dr. Jack Tips

Deep nutritional insights from the ordinary auto-chem, smac-26/CBC blood work.

For the clinical nutritionist, this manual and desk reference examines each blood test value from the SMAC-26/CBC lab test for its nutritional health implications and provides Systemic Formulas protocols for correcting imbalances. Includes optimal values, pathologies, clinical notes, cross references, protocols and valuable insights from other clinicians. An absolutely essential tool for the practicing health professional.

123 pages, ISBN 0-929167-07-4 $44.95

Dragon Rising: Clinician's Guide to the Systemic Chinese Constitutional Formulas by Tena Scarber, LAc and Dr. Jack Tips

In the late 1980's, Doc Wheelwright created the Systemic Chinese Five-Element herbal formulas to address people's constitutional and emotional states. Based on the historic Chinese tradition and the Kempo applications, he perfected the bio-energetic impact of time-honored constitutional herbology and opened up a deeper dimension to herbal healing. This book, a collaborative effort by Jack Tips (Wheelwright Legacy) and Tena Scarber (Acupuncturist), first teaches the Chinese Five-Element foundation and progresses into the unique Wheelwright perspective of bio-energetic correction of fundamental imbalances to create a system of clinical applications to improve the impact of any herbal/nutrition program.

Practitioners who learn to address a patient's constitutional state are able to provide a deeper, more efficient healing directive to help the body adapt and establish its optimal health expression. This material includes the Wheelwright Healing System, formula application triads, formula ingredient discussion, and clinical repertory.

150 pages, illustrations, ISBN #0-929167-29-5, $22.95

SCLEROLOGY / FOOT GLYPHOLOGY

Insights in the Eyes: An Introduction to Sclerology by Dr. Jack Tips

Once you know these 30 signs in the whites of the eye, you have profound insights about a person's constitution and the chief factors that can limit health.

A brief but thorough introduction to the history, premises, and practice of interpreting the red lines in the white of the eyes for stress patterns and nutritional implications. Features the 30 most common stress lines, commentaries, and excerpts from the ISI *Art & Science of Sclerology* Certification Course. A great way to get acquainted with reading the eyes.

70 pages. Illustrations, photos, $19.95

The Art & Science of Sclerology Certification Course by Dr. Jack Tips

Red lines in the whites of your eyes—what do they mean? Here's the most accurate, most advanced, most comprehensive, and most simple training in Sclerology—the interpretation of the red lines in the whites of the eyes for their health implications!

You can become a Sclerologist! Red lines in the whites of your eyes—what do they mean? Here is the most advanced, comprehensive, and up-to-date information in the world on the interpretation of the red lines in the white of the eyes for their health implications. This course will certify you to interpret what the sclera—the whites of the eyes—is revealing about a person's health. This is the International Sclerology Institute's (ISI's) distance education certification course and is the definitive and foundational course for all Sclerologists around the world. Straight from the founder— A.S. Doc Wheelwright, compiled by his protégé, Dr. Jack Tips—this course teaches you to master the stories the eyes can tell. This course communicates the universal language of the eyes. It contains 7-hours of instructional video (tapes CDs) along with a segment on the adrenal glands taught by Wheelwright; a 300-page manual, a full color laminated wall chart; an acetate overlay system to assist practitioners in charting; and the certification examination. Upon successful completion of the course, your certificate will be issued by the ISI and you will be certified as a Sclerologist. More information is on the web site www.sclerology-institute.org.

6-DVD's, 300-page hardback manual with hundreds of color photos, 4-color chart, organ depicting chart, calligraphic pen, acetate overlay charting system, exam, *Insights In the Eyes* book. [List $799] Now $599.

Sclerology Wall Chart by the International Sclerology Institute

The official, international chart of reflex zones in the white of the eyes.

Sclerology is the art of evaluating the entire body's health stresses from the reflexive red lines in the white of the eyes. This is the most accurate and up-to-date chart available. Chart outlines all the reflex zones and demonstrates the line-alphabet.

Artfully designed, four color, 11″ x 17″, laminated, grommets. $29.95

Source Sclerology by the International Sclerology Institute

Come join Doc Wheelwright in this "historic classic" as he teaches Sclerology to a group of health professionals in 1985. This home movie is the only existing record of Wheelwright teaching the insights of his research and the natural healing principles that helped thousands of people experience better health.

5 DVDs ISBN 0-929167-27-9 $159.00

Causations: Using Sclerology To Clairify Iridology
by Drs. Betty Sue O'Brian & Jack Tips

Causations presents the naturopathic philosophy of the critical importance of discovering the fundamental, constitutional cause of a person's symptom portrait. Features groundbreaking discourses by Dr. Jack Tips including: *Holographic Triangulation*, *The Strength of Knowing Your Modality's Weaknesses*, and *The Vision of Causative, Reflexive Information*. This book presents the reasons why reflexive modalities (Sclerology, Iridology) are not diagnostically accurate, but provide even more valuable insights—the *causative* insights. Betty Sue O'Brian provides six case histories, documented with photos, on how Sclerology solved the riddle of a client's case and pointed the way to curative therapy. This book is "a must" for anyone practicing or learning Iridology or Sclerology, as well as for any natural health practitioner who wishes to delve deeper into the body's healing mysteries.

108 pages, ISBN 0-929167-32-5 $21.95

Foot Glyphology by Dr. Jack Tips

The *Foot Glyphology* certification course is the unique, world-definitive modality to interpret the fine lines in the soles of the feet for their health implications direct from the founder, A.S. "Doc" Wheelwright. The soles of the feet provide a critically important insight to Wheelwright's amazing system for understanding the body's inherent struggle to maintain optimal health. He found that the feet often held the determining "hidden causes" behind a person's health concerns-particularly if pathogens such as parasites, bacteria, and fungus were involved. He developed this unique system of 'dermataglyphics' (interpreting the fine lines on the skin) and refined it to its present state in 1989. Wheelwright used the soles' information to 1) gain new insights about tissues in distress, 2) determine if pathogens were involved, 3) validate and differentiate his findings from his sclera analysis, 4) prioritize treatments. This information has never before been published-until now. Includes everything you need to master the interpretation of the lines in the soles of the feet-manual, DVD classroom session, charts, wall chart, exam.

ISBN 0-929167-31-7 [List $399.] Now $299.

Made in the USA
Las Vegas, NV
10 November 2026

57843123R00103